GOLD

LEARN, R
TO GET A HIGHER

- ☑ All official ADA* topics covered in detail
- ☑ Chapter Checklists: Ensure that you meet
  learning objectives
- ☑ Reading Comprehension (RC) strategies a
  techniques to improve your DAT RC score
- ☑ Over 150 practice questions with helpful
- ☑ Free online forum to discuss any chapter
- ☑ This book is 99.9% error-free!

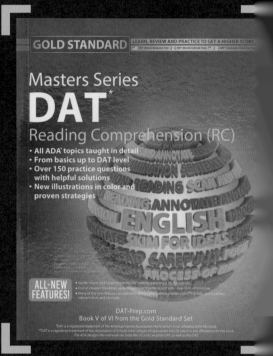

GOLD STANDARD LEARN, REVIEW AND PRACTICE TO GET A HIGHER SCORE

Masters Series
DAT*
Reading Comprehension (RC)

- **All ADA* topics taught in detail**
- **From basics up to DAT level**
- **Over 150 practice questions with helpful solutions**
- **New illustrations in color and proven strategies**

ALL-NEW FEATURES!

DAT-Prep.com
Book V of VI from the Gold Standard Set

*DAT is a registered trademark of the American Dental Association (ADA) which is not affiliated with this book.
**OAT is a registered trademark of the Association of Schools and Colleges of Optometry (ASCO) which is not affiliated with this book.
The ADA designs the real exam for both the US and Canadian DAT, as well as the OAT.

ADA* Official Topics (syllabus: US DAT, Canadian D

"The Reading Comprehension Test contains three reading passages on var
topics. Prior understanding of the science topics is not a prerequisite to a
test items. The reading passages require the ability to read, comprehend, a
analyze basic scientific information."

The DAT Reading Comprehension in a Nutshell

Time allotted for the Section	Total number of questions	Number of passages	Length per passage	Sc Te
60 minutes	**50**	**3**	**1,500** words 9 to 22 numbered paragraphs	in s Hu

DAT-prep.com: Home of Gold Standard DA

The Gold Standard Team of authors and editors includes professi
advanced academic degrees in dentistry, medicine, and the arts, a
League dental students with exceptional DAT scores.

© RuveneCo Inc.

*DAT is a registered trademark of the American Dental Association (ADA) which is not affiliated

The Gold Standard DAT was built for the US DAT.

The Gold Standard DAT is identical to Canadian DAT prep <u>except</u> QR and ORG. Also, you must practice soap carving for the complete Canadian DAT.

The Gold Standard DAT is identical to OAT prep <u>except</u> PAT, which is replaced by OAT Physics; see our Gold Standard OAT book for Physics review and OAT practice test.

Be sure to register at www.DAT-prep.com by clicking on GS DAT Owners and following the directions for Gold Standard DAT Owners. Please Note: benefits are for 1 year from the date of online registration, for the original book owner only and are not transferable; unauthorized access and use outside the Terms of Use posted on DAT-prep.com may result in account deletion; if you are not the original owner, you can purchase your virtual access card separately at DAT-prep.com.

Visit The Gold Standard's Education Center at www.gold-standard.com.

Copyright © 2022 Gold Standard Multimedia Education (Worldwide), DAT Masters Series: Reading Comprehension (RC)

ISBN 978-1-927338-49-0

Address all inquiries, comments, or suggestions to the publisher. For Terms of Use go to: www.DAT-prep.com

RuveneCo Inc
Gold Standard Multimedia Education
559-334 Cornelia St
Plattsburgh, NY 12901
E-mail: learn@gold-standard.com
Online at www.gold-standard.com

DAT™ is a registered trademark of the American Dental Association (ADA). OAT™ is a registered trademark of the Association of Schools and Colleges of Optometry (ASCO). The Dental Aptitude Test (DAT) program is conducted by the Canadian Dental Association (CDA). Ruveneco Inc and Gold Standard Multimedia Education are neither sponsored nor endorsed by the ADA, ASCO, CDA, nor any of the degree granting institutions that the authors have attended or are attending. Printed in China.

The Dental Admission Test (DAT) consists of 280 multiple-choice questions distributed across quite a diversity of question types in four tests. The DAT is a computer-based test (CBT). This exam requires approximately five hours to complete - including the optional tutorial, break, and post-test survey. The following are the four subtests of the Dental Admission Test:

1. **Survey of the Natural Sciences (NS) – 100 questions; 90 min.**
   - General Biology (BIO): 40 questions
   - General Chemistry (CHM): 30 questions
   - Organic Chemistry (ORG): 30 questions

2. **Perceptual Ability Test (PAT) - 90 questions; 6 subsections; 60 min.**
   - Apertures: 15 questions
   - View Recognition: 15 questions
   - Angle Discrimination: 15 questions
   - Paper Folding: 15 questions
   - Cube Counting: 15 questions
   - 3-D Form Development: 15 questions

3. **Reading Comprehension (RC) – 50 questions; 3 reading passages; 60 min.**

4. **Quantitative Reasoning (QR) – 40 questions; 45 min.**
   - Mathematics Problems: 30 questions
   - Applied Mathematics/Word Problems: 10 questions

> **You will get six scores from:**
> (1) BIO (2) CHM (3) ORG (4) PAT (5) QR (6) RC.
>
> **You will get two additional scores which are summaries:**
> (7) Academic Average (AA) = BIO + CHM + ORG + QR + RC
> (8) Total Science (TS) = BIO + CHM + ORG

Common Formula for Acceptance:

GPA + DAT score + Interview = Dental School Admissions*

Figure 1: Typical Overall DAT Score Distribution (Approx.); No. of Test Administrations Annually = 13 000 (Approx.)

*Note: In general, Dental School Admissions Committees will only examine the DAT score if the GPA is high enough; they will only admit or interview if the GPA + DAT score is high enough. Some programs also use autobiographical materials and/or references in the admissions process. Different dental schools may emphasize different aspects of your DAT score, for example: PAT, BIO, TS, AA. The average score for any section is approximately 19/30; the average AA for admissions is usually 18-21 depending on the dental school; the AA for admissions to Harvard is around 23-24; the 100th percentile is usually 25 meaning that virtually 100% of the approximately 13,000 students who take the DAT every year have an AA less than 25. Only a handful of students score 25/30. Our two student contributors scored 27/30 (AA).

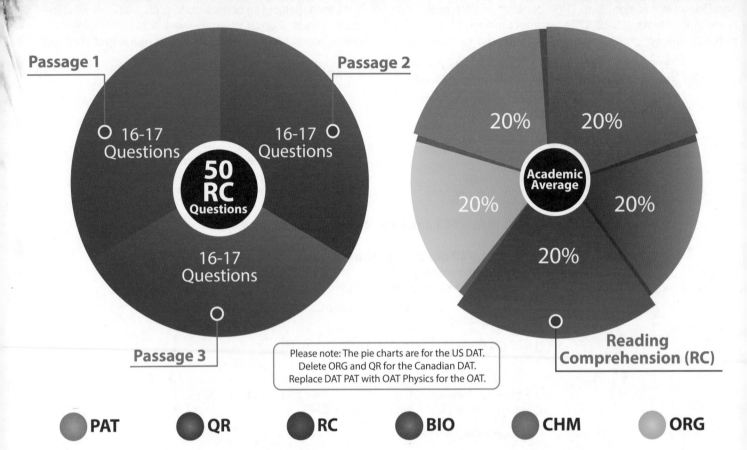

Passage 1 — 16-17 Questions

Passage 2 — 16-17 Questions

50 RC Questions

Passage 3 — 16-17 Questions

Academic Average

20% 20% 20% 20% 20%

Reading Comprehension (RC)

Please note: The pie charts are for the US DAT. Delete ORG and QR for the Canadian DAT. Replace DAT PAT with OAT Physics for the OAT.

● PAT   ● QR   ● RC   ● BIO   ● CHM   ● ORG

The DAT is challenging, get organized.
dat-prep.com/dat-study-schedule

1. How to study
- Learn, review and practice using the DAT Masters Series book(s) and/or videos.
- Complete all exercises and multiple-choice practice questions in this book.
- Consolidate: create and study from your personal summaries (= Gold Notes) daily and/or Anki (*free online flashcards including DAT "Feralis" notes*).

2. Once you have completed your studies
- Complete a full-length DAT practice test.
- Analyze mistakes and all answers/explanations.
- Consolidate: Review all your Gold Notes and create more, with or without Anki.

3. Full-length practice tests
- Take multiple DAT practice tests (varied sources).
- ADA practice exams: Currently, the 2007 exam is free but the most recent exam is paid.
- Free full-length Gold Standard (GS) mock exam GS-Free with helpful, detailed worked solutions.
- Consider other GS or third practice tests if needed.

4. How much time do you need to study?
- On average, 3-6 hours per day for 3-6 months; depending on life experiences, 2 weeks may be enough and 8 months could be insufficient.
- Try to study 'full throttle' for 1-2 weeks and then adjust your expectations for the required time.

5. Recommended DAT Communities
- Although Reddit has a DAT forum, by far, the most active DAT forum on the net is by the Student Doctor Network (SDN): forums.studentdoctor.net/forums/dat-discussions.70/
- Of course, if you have any questions about the content in this book, access for free: dat-prep.com/forum

Is there something in the Masters Series that you did not understand? Don't get frustrated, get online:
dat-prep.com/forum

Table of Contents

DAT-Prep.com

READING
COMPREHENSION

Understand

* Key concepts in academic reading,
  question types, study reading strategies

DAT-Prep.com

Introduction ▮▮▮▮

The DAT Reading Comprehension (RC) entails two main tasks: **(1)** locating key information in academic texts and **(2)** identifying concepts in order to make reasonable inferences about the subject under discussion. These require certain skills that some candidates may already have while others may still need to develop.

In any case, your first step in confronting this section is to familiarize yourself with the features and structure of the test. This will help you determine the approach that you need to adopt in your RC preparation.

Let's start reading!

Multimedia Resources at DAT-Prep.com

Free Online Forum

1.1 Overview

The third section of the DAT is the **Reading Comprehension Test**. This section primarily assesses your ability to locate key details and infer fundamental concepts in scholarly texts. Recall and analysis of written information are skills that are requisite to the problem-solving demands in the basic sciences. Thus the stimulus passages given in the Reading Comprehension section replicate the kind of scientific reading required in dental college.

Prior knowledge of science topics and concepts is NOT REQUIRED to competently answer the test questions, and the best preparation really is, well...reading. However, it is regular study reading from a variety of academic references throughout your high-school and undergraduate studies that makes for a strong foundation in this section. Nevertheless, you should not neglect to prepare for this test as it accounts for one of the five standard scores that make up the Academic Average score in the DAT.

In a report published by the ADA over a decade ago, 39 of the 58 surveyed U.S. dental schools indicated that they consider the Reading Comprehension Test as the third most important DAT score of an applicant, following the Academic Average and Total Science scores, in their admissions criteria.[1] Half of the 10 Canadian dental schools likewise include this score in the DAT, next to Perceptual Ability and Academic Average, as a significant factor in their selection process.

By acquainting yourself with the nature and scope of this section, you will be able to anticipate vulnerable areas. As long as you are quick to address your weaknesses, increasing your chances of doing well in this section is very much possible.

---

[1] ADA Survey Center, *2009-10 Survey of Dental Education Tuition, Admission, and Attrition Volume 2* (Chicago, Illinois: American Dental Association, 2011), http://www.ada.org/sections/professionalResources/pdfs/survey_ed_vol2.pdf.

1.2 Format and Content of the Test

The Reading Comprehension Test is composed of 50 multiple-choice questions and has a time limit of 60 minutes. It consists of three reading passages of approximately 1,500 words in length.

This section comes right after the optional 30-minute break subsequent to the Perceptual Ability Test. A passage is then presented on the computer screen in full-page view. {Please note that the Canadian

DAT remains a paper test and is 50 minutes long. The Reading Comprehension Test is only included in the English DAT in Canada.}

The subsequent screens will show one question at a time, with the reading passage in a parallel window right under it. Every time the page moves to the next question, the reading passage reloads and goes back to its beginning sentence or paragraph.

The DAT is an online test with many features. There is a highlighter tool which you can use to highlight parts of the question and also parts of the reading passage. The highlighted portion will remain on the passage for every question. There is a crossing out tool (~~STRIKEOUT~~), which you can use to cross out answer choices you want to eliminate. Lastly, there is a "MARK" button that you can click to mark a question for yourself to indicate that you want to revisit the question if you have extra time.

The Reading Passage

A passage is placed in a smaller window with a vertical scroll bar that allows the test-taker to move the text up and down. Paragraphs are also numbered. The "NEXT" button at the bottom-center of the window leads to the questions in the succeeding pages.

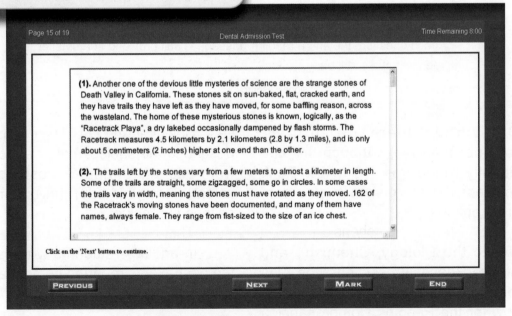

Page 15 of 19 — Dental Admission Test — Time Remaining 8:00

(1). Another one of the devious little mysteries of science are the strange stones of Death Valley in California. These stones sit on sun-baked, flat, cracked earth, and they have trails they have left as they have moved, for some baffling reason, across the wasteland. The home of these mysterious stones is known, logically, as the "Racetrack Playa", a dry lakebed occasionally dampened by flash storms. The Racetrack measures 4.5 kilometers by 2.1 kilometers (2.8 by 1.3 miles), and is only about 5 centimeters (2 inches) higher at one end than the other.

(2). The trails left by the stones vary from a few meters to almost a kilometer in length. Some of the trails are straight, some zigzagged, some go in circles. In some cases the trails vary in width, meaning the stones must have rotated as they moved. 162 of the Racetrack's moving stones have been documented, and many of them have names, always female. They range from fist-sized to the size of an ice chest.

Click on the 'Next' button to continue.

PREVIOUS   NEXT   MARK   END

Figure RC.1.1: Screenshot of a Reading Passage.

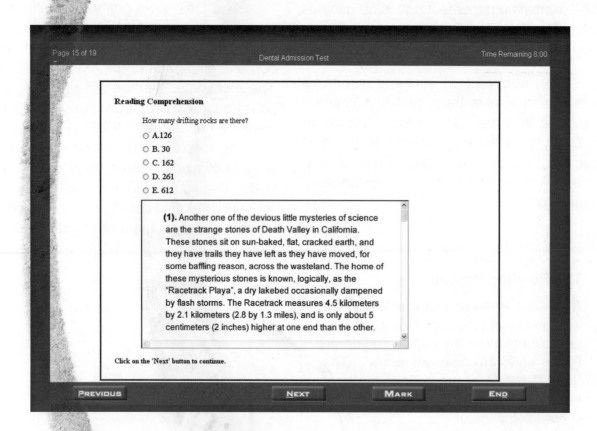

Figure RC.1.2: Screen Window View of the Questions. Take note that for each question, the entire reading passage is still provided in a smaller screen with the scroll bar.

On average, there are 16 to 17 questions per passage, although this can occasionally range from 15 to 20. Each question requires an answer choice from four to five options.

Unlike the Biology, Chemistry and Quantitative Reasoning sections, the ADA has not published any recommended text to review for the Reading Comprehension Test. However, the DAT User's Manual has described the subject matter as "developed from aspects of dental, basic, or clinical science not covered in an undergraduate college curriculum."

In addition, students who have taken the past exams reported coming across the following topics:

Science Topics

- Aging
- Antibiotics
- Bone fractures
- Brain functions, glutamate receptors
- Contraception
- Einstein-related topic
- Enzymes, telomerases
- Fungi
- Gene therapy, genetic cancer, epithelial-mesenchymal transition

- Helico bacteria (H.Pylori)
- Herbal medicine
- Hurricanes
- Physics involving calculations
- Subatomic particles
- Tooth development
- Transcription/Translation, recent studies on mRNA, voltage-gated ion channels, messenger

Non-science topics

- Ethics
- Floating Bridges

- Piano
- The Stock Market

Please note that you do neither have to know nor study these topics in order to do well on the exam. Rather, these merely serve as examples to give you a glimpse of the subject matters typically found on the test.

The DAT Reading Comprehension in a Nutshell				
Time allotted for the Section	Total number of questions	Number of passages	Length per passage	Topics
60 minutes	**50**	**3**	**1,500** words 9 to 22 numbered paragraphs	Scientific and Technical in some instances Humanities

Understand

* Reading comprehension techniques: predicting, skimming, paraphrasing, visualizing, contextual clues

DAT-Prep.com

Introduction ▮▮▮▮

Questions in the DAT Reading Comprehension Test mostly require careful attention to specific terms, methods and/or core ideas in a passage. On some occasions, you may need to slow down and evaluate certain details with an analytical perspective.

Reading techniques such as predicting, skimming, and paraphrasing should form the backbone of your preparation. The earlier you utilize these skills, the earlier you will be able to identify which strategies are the most effective for you.

Multimedia Resources at DAT-Prep.com

Free Online Forum

2.1 Factors Affecting Preparation and Performance in the Test

In the preceding chapter, we have discussed the format and content of the DAT Reading Comprehension Test.

Knowing what to expect in this section is quite important because the difficulty of a test is oftentimes subjective to the test-taker. For instance, some passages may appear lengthy because paragraphs in the RC section are numbered, making short but several paragraphs look longer. Being confronted with a seemingly lengthy passage may set an anxious examinee to panic, consequentially affecting focus and confidence in overcoming the whole test.

However, if you very well know beforehand that a reading passage will only have 1500 words at the maximum, and assuming that you have adequately practiced your reading speed for this section, you can calmly proceed with the exam.

Likewise, the difficulty of a specific passage depends on a candidate's background. Someone who is not used to reading dense articles whether in the sciences or humanities often find the RC section a real challenge. Moreover, humanities in the DAT RC context specifically refer to philosophical texts that deal with moral values or socio-political principles. Readings based on culture or the arts are also common. A student with a strong science background may find these readings difficult because of limited exposure to such topics.

Applicants who have English as their second language doubly struggle in the RC section because the language used in these passages is largely technical.

Building your skills effectively for this section indeed depends on a number of factors. However, familiarity with science topics, exposure to technical and scholarly reading, timing and the ability to focus are all key components to success. While no specific presumed knowledge is required to answer any of the questions, you still need to remain focused on cultivating these core skills, which will be tested in the actual exam.

2.2 Developing Comprehension Skills

2.2.1 One Year or More before the DAT

Strengthening your reading comprehension skills is beneficial to your overall preparation for the DAT: you are more likely to overcome better the cognitive rigor of the different test sections. By exposing yourself to various topics, your stored knowledge will also expand. This will be particularly important when you start interviewing for dental school and present yourself as a well-rounded individual.

Therefore, read! Be known as a "voracious reader"! Read materials that interest you, as well as those that DO NOT necessarily excite you. After all, dental school involves a lot of reading and absorbing enormous amounts of information.

Contrary to approaching creative and opinion pieces, some extent of background knowledge makes reading scientific articles a less agonizing experience. You tend to understand technical concepts better and quicker if you have been introduced to the topic before. At least once every week, for 1 – 3 hours, you should read among the following (either from a university library or online):

● **Scientific Articles**

Suggested Resources:

✓ **Dental Journals**
The Journal of the American Dental Association (http://jada.ada.org/)
The Journal of Contemporary Dental Practice (http://www.thejcdp.com/)
Journal of Dental Research (http://jdr.sagepub.com/)
The Directory of Open Access Journals (http://www.doaj.org/) This free-access site lists the links to online dental journals.

✓ **Dental Research and News Sources**
Pubmed has several articles that have free Full Text content: http://www.ncbi.nlm.nih.gov/pubmed/
ADA Science News (http://ada.org/272.aspx)
ADA Publications and Resources (http://ada.org/293.aspx)

✓ **Science Magazines**
The Scientific American (http://www.scientificamerican.com/sciammag/)
Discover Magazine (http://discovermagazine.com/)

Active reading tends to improve comprehension and speed. With scientific articles, the following techniques usually prove to be helpful:

1. **Predicting**

   This is equivalent to preliminary skimming. Upon seeing the title of what you are about to read, you can usually guess the article's content, especially if you are familiar with the subject matter from prior knowledge. Likewise, awareness of textual types (e.g., expository*, argumentative) could help predict to which the succeeding discussions may lead.

2. **Skimming**

   This is a technique for spotting clues within the text itself. You run your eyes quickly through the content for an overview of what to expect in the material, occasionally slowing down on seemingly salient parts. As you skim over the words and the paragraphs, you should continually ask yourself…

   - Is this article about a description of some characteristic?
   - Is the article about an origin, a discovery or a scientific process or method?

- Does the author organize his or her ideas through definitions and examples, classification, or cause and effect?

   By using this technique, you can figure out certain parts that are not essential and detect parts where you need to dedicate some attention for a better understanding of the details. Lastly, skimming will confirm your earlier prediction, which was initially based on the article's title.

3. **Paraphrasing**

   In order to test your general understanding of reading material, restate the main idea of each relevant paragraph. By the end of the article, you will have a clearer outline of the author's central point. Taking the whole by its smaller parts is less overwhelming than having to swallow everything in a single glance.

4. **Visualizing**

   Quite frequently, the procedures and the apparatus described in scientific papers are very specific. For descriptions of the parts of an instrument, doing a sketch proves to be of great benefit. Similarly, you can create a skeletal outline of the steps in an experiment, a research investigation, or a process.

---

*Expository texts can range from textbooks to scientific journals, encyclopedia, and biographies. These articles are meant to inform, describe, explain or define concepts, theories and methods.

- **Humanities Articles**

For exposure to a variety of the humanities topics and themes, include Arts and Culture articles in your weekly plate of exploratory reading:

✓ **Humanities and Culture Magazines or Journals**
The New Yorker - Culture section (http://www.newyorker.com/arts/)
Digital Humanities (http://www.digitalhumanities.org/dhq/)
The Culture Magazine (http://www.culturemachine.net/)

Paraphrasing is a reading technique that is highly applicable to selections from the humanities and any texts that demand inference. However, you should go beyond just getting the main idea. The following are also vital questions that you need to actively ask yourself when reading non-scientific articles:

- What are the primary supporting facts and/or evidences that support the author's thesis?
- For which type of audience would the article appeal?
- What is the author's tone?
- What is the author's attitude or opinion toward the subject?
- What is the author's purpose for writing the article?

2.3 One Year or Less before the DAT

Read section 2.2.1 one more time! Even at this point in your preparation, being a voracious reader - with all that it entails - should be your goal. Besides reading, you need to practice.

The best strategy is to take the ADA's *DAT Sample Test Items*, which can be downloaded for free from the ADA website. Although this is not a full-length test, you should still do this section within the prescribed time limit (approximately 1.2 minutes per question). Your main objective is to gauge your current skills against the requirements of the real test. You should be able to determine this by reviewing your mistakes.

If you performed well and understood the source of your errors then you will only require ADA and the Gold Standard (GS) DATs in order to complete your preparation. If, on the other hand, you struggled in the test or struggled to understand your mistakes then you may need additional work on strategies, practice or a formal course for or without credit. An optional RC program can be found at DAT-prep.com.

Basic Preparation Tools	Practice Exams (Full-length)
• ADA *DAT Sample Items* • Your Masters Series DAT RC book	• DAT Practice Test (ADA) • Masters Series DAT PAT book (GS-1) or GS exams online • Third party practice tests (free or paid)

2.4 Advice for ESL Students

The same preparation applies for candidates with English as a second language (ESL). Depending on your English skills, you may or may not benefit from an English reading or writing summer course. Of course, you would have the option of deciding whether or not you would want to take such a course for credit.

However, vocabulary may be a chief obstacle, so getting used to academic and rhetorical language is imperative. The dictionary will have to be a constant help buddy in the beginning; but as you progress in your speed and vocabulary, you need to wean yourself from the dictionary and start counting on context clues.

2.5 Contextual Reading

Contextual reading compels you to make a logical guess about the meaning of an unknown word based on the other words and phrases found within the immediate sentences in the paragraph. Writers themselves use this technique to make lucid points. Several cues easily offer probable definitions to uncommon terms:

1) Examples
Cue words: includes, consists of, such as

Equine animals, such as horses and zebras, have long been used not only to aid in man's work but also to assist in therapy.

Using the example clue (use of "such as"), the word equine means:

A. *mammal.*
B. *reptile.*
C. *horse group.*
D. *dog.*

2) Synonyms
   Cue words: is similar to, just as, also means

   *Calling my cousin an "eccentric weirdo" is **tautologous**! It is similar to telling a ghost that he is dead twice.*

   The cue word "is similar to" indicates that tautologous means:

A. *repetitive.*
B. *alien.*
C. *scary.*
D. *ridiculous.*

3) Antonyms and Contrasts
   Cue words: unlike, contrary to/in contrast, on the other hand, as opposed to

   *Contrary to the playwright's **euphemisms** about the King's corrupt leadership, the merchant was quite direct in criticizing the latter's injustices.*

   Based on the contrasting descriptions used in the sentence, the word euphemism refers to:

A. *corruption.*
B. *indirect speech.*
C. *criticism.*
D. *politics.*

Answers:
1. C
2. A
3. B

Rules about upside down answers: As a rule, if answers are on the same page or on a page facing the questions, the answers will be upside down to avoid distraction (*or cheating??*)! Answers are not upside down if they are *au verso* (on the back page of the questions). As long as it is for personal use, you can take a pic with your smartphone and rotate to more conveniently read the answers. If you are using the DAT-prep.com eBook reader, you also have the option of using the rotation function.

4) Sense of the sentence

Oftentimes, you only need to observe how the words or phrases relate within the sentence in order to fairly conclude what the difficult word means. Take careful note of the descriptions in the paragraph. Use your logic in determining the most probable meaning of a newly-encountered term.

March 21, 1894 marks a rare series of **syzygies** *in the history of astronomical events. A few hours before Mercury transits the sun as seen from Venus, a partial lunar eclipse is witnessed from Earth. From Saturn, both Mercury and Venus could be seen simultaneously transiting the sun. Such planetary spectacles can also be observed by the naked human eye during full moons and new moons as the sun, our planet Earth, and the moon periodically aligns.*

Based on the context of the discussion in the paragraph, the closest meaning of syzygies could be:

A. *planetary collisions.*
B. *lunar eclipses.*
C. *planetary alignments.*
D. *historical changes.*

5) Root Words, Prefixes, and Suffixes

Certain root words and word parts carry specific meanings. Being acquainted with these, combined with the other clues discussed earlier, helps you figure out the most probable meaning of an unfamiliar word.

Answer: C

Descriptions in the paragraph mention "lunar eclipse," "Mercury transits the sun," and "the sun, our planet earth, and the moon periodically aligns." These should serve as primary clues in determining a general definition of syzygies.

(D) Historical changes is obviously the least likely option. (A) Planetary collisions may sound related; however, nothing in the paragraph indicates a collision of the planets. This should now narrow down your choice between (B) lunar eclipses and (C) planetary alignments. Now common knowledge tells us that a lunar eclipse occurs when three celestial bodies such as the sun, the moon and the Earth align. On the other hand, a full moon or a new moon does not necessarily result to a lunar eclipse. This makes C the more logical answer!

2.6 Common Root Words of Scientific Terms

The following is a list of root words, prefixes, and suffixes, which you would generally find in scientific literature. A prefix is a group of letters added to the beginning of a word; a suffix is added to the end of a word. If you find this section helpful for your RC (or even DAT BIO) prep, consider reading the prefixes and suffixes into an MP3 file on your smartphone which you can listen to while exercising, waiting in line, or during daily transportation as your scheduled DAT approaches.

Prefixes

A
aden- gland
adip- fat
aero- air
agri- field; soil
alb- white
alg-/algia- pain
alto- high
ambi- both
ameb- change; alternation
amni- fetal membrane
amphi-; ampho- both
amyl- starch
ana- up; back; again
andro- man; masculine
anemo- wind
angi- blood vessel; duct
ante- before; ahead of time
anter- front
antho- flower
anthropo- man; human
aqu- water
archaeo- primitive; ancient
arteri- artery
arthr- joint; articulation

aster-; astr- ; astro- star
ather- fatty deposit
atmo- vapor
audi- hear
aur- ear
auto- self

B
bacter-/bactr- bacterium; stick; club
baro- weight
bath- depth; height
bene- well; good
bi- (Latin) two; twice
bi-/bio- (Greek) life; living
brachi- arm
brachy- short
brady- slow
branchi- fin
bronch- windpipe

C
calor- heat
capill- hair
capit- head
carcin- cancer

Prefixes

cardi-/cardio- heart
carn- meat; flesh
carp- fruit
carpal- wrist
cata- breakdown; downward
caud- tail
cente- pierce
centi- hundredth
centr- center
cephal- head
cerat- horn
cerebr- brain
cervic- neck
chel- claw
chem- dealing with chemicals
chir- hand
chlor- green
chondr- cartilage
chrom-/chromo- color
chron- time
circa-; circum- around; about
cirru- hairlike curls
co- with; together
cocc- seed; berry
coel- hollow
coll- glue
coni- cone
contra- against
corp- body
cort-/cortic- outer layer
cosmo- world; order; form
cotyl- cup
counter- against
crani- skull

cresc-/cret- begin to grow
crypt- hidden; covered
cumul- heaped
cuti- skin
cyt- cell; hollow container

D
dactyl- finger
deca- ten
deci- tenth
deliquesc- become fluid
demi- half
dendr- tree
dent- tooth
derm- skin
di-/dipl- (Latin) two; double
di-/dia- (Greek) through; across; apart
dia- (Latin) day
digit- finger; toe
din- terrible
dis- apart; out
dorm- sleep
dors- back
du-/duo- two
dynam- power
dys- bad; abnormal; difficult

E
ec- out of; away from
echin- spiny; prickly
eco- house
ecto- outside of
en-/endo-/ent- in; into; within
encephal- brain

Prefixes

enter- intestine; gut
entom- insects
epi- upon; above; over
erythro- red
eso- inward; within; inner

F
ferro- iron
fibr- fiber; thread
fiss- split
flor- flower
flu-; fluct-; flux flow
foli- leaf
fract- break

G
gastr- stomach
geo- land; earth
gloss- tongue
gluc-/glyc- sweet; sugar
glut- buttock
gnath- jaw
gymno- naked; bare
gyn- female
gyr- ring; circle; spiral

H
halo- salt
hapl- simple
hecto- hundred
hem- blood
hemi- half
hepar/hepat- liver
herb- grass; plants

hetero- different; other
hex- six
hibern- winter
hidr- sweat
hipp- horse
hist- tissue
holo- entire; whole
homo- (Latin) man; human
homo- (Greek) same; alike
hort- garden
hydr- water
hygr- moist; wet
hyper- above; beyond; over
hyph- weaving; web
hypno- sleep
hypo- below; under; less
hyster- womb; uterus

I
ichthy- fish
infra- below; beneath
inter- between
intra- within; inside
iso- equal; same

K
kel- tumor; swelling
kerat- horn
kilo- thousand
kine- move

L
lachry- tear
lact- milk

Prefixes

lat- side
leio- smooth
leuc-/leuk- white; bright; light
lign- wood
lin- line
lingu- tongue
lip- fat
lith-; -lite stone; petrifying
loc- place
lumin- light

M
macr- large
malac- soft
malle- hammer
mamm- breast
marg- border; edge
mast- breast
med- middle
meg- million; great
mela-/melan- black; dark
mes- middle; half; intermediate
met-/meta- between; along; after
micro- small; millionth
milli- thousandth
mis- wrong; incorrect
mito- thread
mole- mass
mono- one; single
mort- death
morph- shape; form
multi- many
mut- change
my- muscle

myc- fungus
mycel- threadlike
myria- many
moll- soft

N
nas- nose
necr- corpse; dead
nemat- thread
neo- new; recent
nephro- kidney
neur- nerve
noct-/nox- night
non- not
not- back
nuc- center

O
ob- against
ocul- eye
oct- eight
odont- tooth
olf- smell
oligo- few; little
omni- all
onc- mass; tumor
opthalm- eye
opt- eye
orb- circle; round; ring
ornith- bird
orth- straight; correct; right
oscu- mouth
oste- bone
oto- ear

Prefixes

ov-/ovi- egg
oxy- sharp; acid; oxygen

P
pachy - thick
paleo- old; ancient
palm- broad; flat
pan- all
par-/para- beside; near; equal
path- disease; suffering
pent- five
per- through
peri- around
permea- pass; go
phag- eat
pheno- show
phon- sound
photo- light
phren- mind; diaphragm
phyc- seaweed; algae
phyl- related group
physi- nature; natural qualities
phyt- plant
pino- drink
pinni- feather
plan- roaming; wandering
plasm- formed into
platy- flat
pleur- lung; rib; side
pneumo- lungs; air
poly- many; several
por- opening
port- carry
post- after; behind

pom- fruit
pre- before; ahead of time
prim- first
pro- forward; favoring; before
proto- first; primary
pseudo- false; deceptive
psych- mind
pter- having wings or fins
pulmo- lung
puls- drive; push
pyr- heat; fire

Q
quadr- four
quin- five

R
radi- ray
ren- kidney
ret- net; made like a net
rhe- flow
rhin- nose
rhiz- root
rhodo- rose
roto- wheel
rubr- red

S
sacchar- sugar
sapr- rotten
sarc- flesh
saur- lizard
schis-/schiz- split; divide
sci- know

Prefixes

scler- hard
semi- half; partly
sept- partition; seven
sex- six
sol- sun
solv- loosen; free
som-/somat- body
somn- sleep
son- sound
spec-/spic- look at
spir- breathe
stat- standing; staying
stell- stars
sten- narrow
stern- chest; breast
stom- mouth
strat- layer
stereo- solid; 3-dimensional
strict- drawn tight
styl- pillar
sub- under; below
super-/sur- over; above; on top
sym-/syn- together

T
tachy- quick; swift
tarso- ankle
tax- arrange; put in order
tele- far off; distant
telo- end
terr- earth; land
tetr- four
thall- young shoot

toxico- poison
top- place
trache- windpipe
trans- across
tri- three
trich- hair
turb- whirl

U
ultra- beyond
uni- one
ur- urine

V
vas- vessel
vect- carry
ven-/vent- come
ventr- belly; underside
vig- strong
vit-/viv- life
volv- roll; wander

X
xanth- yellow
xero- dry
xyl- wood

Z
zo- animal
zyg- joined together
zym- yeast

Suffixes

A
-ap/-aph -touch
-ary/-arium -place for something
-ase -forms names of enzymes

B
-blast -sprout; germ; bud

C
-cell -chamber; small room
-chrome -color
-chym -juice
-cid/-cis -cut; kill; fall
-cul/-cule -small; diminutive
-cyst -sac; pouch; bladder
-cyte -cell; hollow container

D
-duct -lead
E
-elle -small
-emia -blood
-en -made of
-eous -nature of; like
-err -wander; go astray

F
-fer -bear; carry; produce
-fid -divided into
-flect/-flex -bend

G
-gam -marriage
-gene -origin; birth

-gest -carry; produce; bear
-glen -eyeball
-glob -ball; round
-gon -angle; corner

H
-hal/-hale -breathe; breath
-helminth -worm

I
-iac -person afflicted with disease
-iasis -disease; abnormal condition
-ism -a state or condition
-ist -person who deals with...
-itis -inflammation; disease
-ium -refers to a part of the body

K
-kary -cell nucleus

L
-less -without
-log -word; speech
-logist -one who studies...
-logy -study of...
-lys/-lyt/-lyst -decompose; split; dissolve

M
-mer -part
-meter/-metry measurement
-mot -move

Suffixes

N
-ner -moist; liquid
-node -knot
-nom/-nomy -ordered knowledge; law

O
-oid -form; appearance
-oma -abnormal condition; tumor
-orium/-ory -place for something
-osis -abnormal condition

P
-pathy -disease; suffering
-ped -foot
-ped -child
-phil -loving; fond of
-phone -sound
-phore; pher -bear; carry
-phyll -leaf
-phyte -plant
-plast -form
-pod -foot

R
-rrhage -burst forth
-rrhea -flow

S
-scop -look; device for seeing
-septic -infection; putrefaction
-sis -condition; state
-sperm -seed
-spher -ball; round
-spire -breathe
-spor -seed

-stasis -placed
-stome -mouth

T
-the/-thes -put
-thel -cover a surface
-therm -heat
-tom -cut; slice
-trop -turn; change
-troph -nourishment; one who feeds

U
-ul/-ule -diminutive; small
-ura -tail
-verge -turn; slant
-vor -devour; eat

Z
-zoa -animal

Chapter Checklist

☐ Sign up or access your free online account at www.dat-prep.com to join the forum to discuss any content from this chapter or any practice questions in this Masters Series book.

☐ Complete a maximum of 1 page of notes using symbols/abbreviations to represent the entire chapter. These are your Gold Notes.

☐ Consider your options based on your optimal way of learning:

    ☐ Create your own, tangible study cards or try the free app: Anki.

    ☐ Record your voice reading your Gold Notes onto your smartphone (MP3s) and listen during exercise, transportation, etc. (*see RC 2.5 as an example*).

    ☐ Consider reading at least 1 source material every day (*see RC 2.2.1*). Note down the main idea or ideas of the piece on your scratch paper. Determine or surmise the author's sentiment or purpose for writing the material.

☐ Schedule your full-length DAT practice tests: ADA and/or GS exams and/or other free or paid third-party resources. Schedule one full day to complete a practice test and 1-2 days for a thorough assessment of answers and explanations while adding to your abbreviated Gold Notes.

☐ Schedule and/or evaluate stress reduction techniques such as regular exercise (sports), yoga, meditation and/or mindfulness exercises (*see* YouTube for suggestions).

Understand

* DAT-specific exam strategies
  and approaches
* Types of questions

DAT-Prep.com

Introduction

Speed reading is a critical skill in the Reading Comprehension Test. The DAT RC specifically calls for mental endurance and efficiency. For one, this section comes after the Perceptual Ability Test – which can already be mentally exhausting! For another, questions on the DAT RC require you to QUICKLY spot key details, delineate facts from opinion, and as the term "comprehension" implies, understand the central point of the written piece.

In this chapter, we will show you clear and specific strategies and build your skills with dozens of exercises. This will be followed by four separate mini-RC tests and then a full-length practice RC test. Let's begin . . .

Multimedia Resources at DAT-Prep.com

Free Online Forum

3.1 How to Approach the Reading Comprehension Section

Three passages to read – each with approximately 1500 words – and a total of 50 questions to answer in 60 minutes! How do you complete this test on time and ace it?

Indeed, time management poses a major challenge to many test-takers. The DAT RC, however, is not merely about speed reading. This section will also require mental endurance after a demanding one-hour Perceptual Ability Test. Likewise, efficiency in locating relevant information and understanding key ideas are integral factors that will help you overcome the demands of this section.

Nevertheless, students have aced the section using different strategies. There is no "one size fits all" strategy to obtain a great score. The key is to be able to start early with your preparation so you can identify which strategy specifically works for you. A systematic approach with clear strategies – some sort of a game plan – is vital in achieving an excellent RC score.

Ideally, you should make a concerted effort to try the various strategies that we present to you during separate timed practice tests. Then you can compare the various scores which you have obtained. This will help you narrow down the specific strategies that apply to your own experience. From that point onward, you should remain consistent.

> Ample Preparation Time + Clear Strategies + Simulated Practice Tests

3.1.1 Methods in Reading Passages during the Exam

Generally, you would need to read carefully but swiftly. You will have about 20 minutes per passage. Every 30 minutes, you should check the timer on the computer to be sure that you have completed approximately 25 questions. Of course you can judge time in any way you want (20, 25, 30-minute intervals, etc.). But decide on a system during practice and commit to that system on test day.

Be sure to reach a speed where you have at least 10 minutes to spare. If you have time at the end, you can return to properly evaluate the questions you skipped or marked. Of course, if you find that you are getting behind the set pace, then you consistently guess the answers to time-consuming questions in order to catch up.

In the meantime, you should try to apply each of the strategies that we will discuss in this section in order to determine which gives you your optimal performance. Different DAT students have boosted their RC scores with completely different techniques. With constant practice, you will be able to determine which of the following is best for you.

1. Questions First, Passage Once

Some candidates like to get a glimpse of the questions prior to reading the text. Others read the questions but not the answer choices yet. Then they read the passage and answer questions as they read the information. The point of doing this is to survey the kind of reading technique that will work best in attacking the passage and which other strategy to employ.

You may find it more efficient to work in this manner. Try one of the practice exams using this strategy and if you find it easier to answer the questions correctly, you should use the same method on the actual DAT.

2. Passage First, Questions Next

Some examinees prefer to carefully read through the passage once while noting the key details. Remember that the DAT is a computerized exam, and you will be provided with laminated noteboards at your test center upon request. You can take brief notes of the major ideas and concepts in each paragraph along with their keywords. You can use boxes and or circles to categorize the important details and then, make meaningful connections between the main concepts and their supporting information by using arrows. This is also called "mapping."

This strategy allows you to mark significant information in specific paragraphs so that they are easier to locate when answering relevant questions later. At the same time, you can see where the discussion is going as you construct each part of the "map." Ideally, you should be able to make a reasonable conclusion of the author's central thesis once you complete the "map."

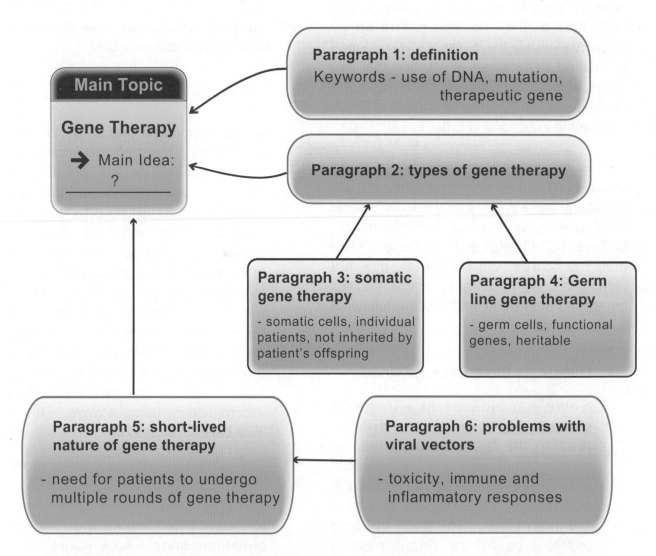

Figure RC 3.1: Mapping a Passage. Start with the main box using the passage's title as the main topic. You can then use circles and boxes to help you categorize the main concepts and their supporting details, respectively. By the time that you complete "mapping" Paragraph 6, you can safely infer that the passage's main idea is roughly about the disadvantages of gene therapy.

3. Questions and Passage at the Same Time

This approach may not always work with questions that greatly require identifying the central idea of a passage. However, for questions that merely ask you to locate data such as dates, names, terminologies or definitions, this exam reading method is time-saving.

You read each question as you proceed with the test, and then skim through the different paragraphs to find the correct answer.

4. Read the Opening and Closing Paragraphs

In many cases, you would need to combine one or two of the preceding approaches in dealing with the passages. Going over the first and last paragraphs of a passage gives you a "bracket" to work within.

Once you get an initial feel of the passage, you can decide on the appropriate strategy that will speed up your performance during the exam.

We have also established that reading diverse material in the period leading up to the exam will be useful since the stimulus material will be from a variety of sources. Create a mindset that, in the exam, you are prepared for "edutainment": After completing a passage, look forward to what you can learn and discover in the next one. Having properly prepared and then begin the exam with the right attitude will give you an edge.

In any case, the most logical means to find out which strategy or which combination of strategies would augment your test-taking skills is to do simulated practice. The more you practice, the more you are inclined to be comfortable with a particular strategy or modify a technique to suit your own strengths or weaknesses.

3.1.2 Basic Question and Answer Techniques

Understanding the "science" of answering multiple choice questions is another vital skill in dealing with not only the Reading Comprehension section, but also with the DAT exam as a whole. The

following are general techniques used in answering such questions.

1. Process of Elimination (PoE): eliminate any answers that are obviously

wrong. In many cases, there may be two very similar answer choices that appear to be correct. You would need to pay close attention to the subtle differences in order to determine the actual answer. Dismissing the obvious ones first from your choices would certainly save you a lot of precious time. If you have second thoughts about your remaining choices, the exam's program allows you to mark an answer so you can go back to it later - if you have enough time left - and decide on your final choice.

2. **Never lose sight of the question:** by the time students read answer choices C and D, some have forgotten the question and are simply looking for "true" sounding statements. Therefore, they tend to choose an option, which presents a statement that may be true but does not answer the question, and is therefore incorrect. For example,

Answer Choice D: Most people are of average height. → This is a true statement.

However, the question was: What is the weight of most people?

Therefore, the true statement becomes the incorrect answer!

Continually check the question and

check or cross out right or wrong answers.

3. **Paying attention to details:** a common decoy in most timed multiple-choice exams, and especially in the DAT RC, is to offer options that are in close proximity – either within the same sentence or paragraph – where the correct answer is found. At other times, either the phrasing of the statements in the answer choices or the language used in the passage itself is complicated. Hence you need to stay focused on the facts and thoroughly understand both the information and the question presented.

EXAMPLE

Question: What is the most effective treatment for OLP?

A. Corrective dentistry
B. Regular dental consultations
C. Systemic corticosteroids
D. Non-randomized clinical trials

Text: Although systemic corticosteroids are probably the most effective treatment modality for patients with diffuse erosive OLP (oral lichen planus) or multi-site disease, the literature on their use is limited to non-randomized clinical trials. Thus oral hygiene and corrective dentistry play a major role in the management of OLP and consultation with a dentist or oral medicine specialist is helpful.

Answer: Getting the facts straight in this test item can be tricky. The question is simply asking for the most effective treatment, regardless of its actual use or availability of helpful alternatives. Thus the correct answer is C.

4. **Verbatim Statements:** Literal and direct quotes from the stimulus material characterize several of the correct answer choices in the real DAT. This is because topics in the reading passages mostly deal with scientific and literal matters.

The next question-and-answer techniques, which we will discuss, are rarely required in the DAT RC. However, these are common "tricks" in multiple choice questions, which are worth getting yourself familiar with – just in case they do come up in the exam.

5. **Beware of the extreme:** words such as always, never, perfect, totally, and completely are often (but not always) clues that the answer choice is incorrect.

6. **Mean Statements:** mean or politically incorrect statements are unlikely to be included in a correct answer choice. For example, if you see any of the following statements in an answer choice, you can pretty much guarantee that it is not the correct answer:

Parents should abuse their children.
Poor people are lazy.
Religion is socially destructive.
Torture is usually necessary.

3.2 DAT-specific RC Exam Strategies

While the preceding methods and techniques are effective in tackling the RC section, there are strategies that specifically address the types of questions presented in the DAT.

1. **Scan and Locate (SaL)**

You will most probably make the most use of this strategy. When you scan, you simply locate specific details that ask the basic "who, what, when, where, and how." Basically, you will be looking for proper nouns and numerical figures. It is similar to browsing the telephone directory to look up an address or contact number.

If you have been practicing the reading techniques recommended in Chapter 2, this strategy might become almost second nature to you. This is probably the easiest skill to develop, yet a very important one. Efficiently locating a specific detail trains you to differentiate material information from immaterial ones; those that add something new from those that simply restate an idea.

Scanning will work even without a preview of the questions. You simply proceed with each question – one at a time – and rapidly find the data being asked by scrolling down and up the passage, then move on to the next. Note the scanned details – either mentally or by writing them down – and remember that these are key to the passage's overall discussion. For example, the answer to a question "Which of the following experiments resulted in the widespread cure of such disease?" must be pertinent to the passage. You can then use this as one of your bases to understand the main idea better or to determine the author's purpose.

2. Skim for Ideas (SI)

The main difference between scanning and skimming is that you search for words or numerical values in the former while sentences and ideas in the latter. Skimming is mostly useful when the information that you are looking for is not explicitly stated in the passage. Therefore, you randomly seek for supporting data, more keywords, examples or explanations. Whenever you find one, slow down and read for the precise information you need.

3. Outline and Annotate (OA)

Outlining is more or less the same as the reading technique "paraphrasing" discussed in Chapter 2. You can use this strategy as a conjunction either after you have shortly gone over the questions or as you go along assessing the passage first. The advantage, on the other hand, of doing an initial glimpse of the different questions is that you get to have a heads-up as to whether the passage will simply require scanning information or demand an in-depth understanding of concepts. In most instances, this strategy tends to work best with inference questions.

Essentially, you jot down key terms and ideas of each numbered paragraph. Please note, however, that the Canadian

DAT does not allow the use of any paper other than the answer sheet provided. For the American DAT, as mentioned earlier, you can ask for a noteboard, which is provided in the test center. Doing so helps you to read actively and then later, to find keywords or points without having to search aimlessly. Your notes can also include any one or more of the following that you deem relevant:

- brief remarks of each paragraph's main idea
- definition of key terms
- hypothetical examples or interpretations of important concepts
- your observations of the author's tone, writing style, attitude toward the subject, or devices used to illustrate a point
- your own questions or doubts

about ambiguous points in the paragraph

Some candidates also find it helpful to do the following: just before you read from each passage, think of someone young that you know - for example, a younger brother, sister, cousin, etc. Imagine that once you finish reading the stimulus material, you will have to explain it to them in words that they understand. The idea is to encourage active reading, attention and focus.

An alternative scenario, if it does not stress you out too much, would be to imagine that you will need to give a speech in class regarding the passage right after you read it once. Keep that imagery during your evaluation of the material, so you have a heightened sense of awareness of what you are reading.

Gold Standard DAT RC Key Methods and Strategies

- Scan and Locate (SaL)
- Skim for Ideas (SI)
- Outline and Annotate (OA)
- Process of Elimination (PoE)
- Attention to Details
- Never lose sight of the question

3.3 Types of Questions

Questions in the DAT Reading Comprehension section can be loosely classified into two main categories: detail-oriented and concept-oriented.

1. Detail-oriented

Questions of this type chiefly test your accurate identification of facts or key concepts found in the passage.

A. Recall Questions

You will need to search the passage for terms, synonyms, proper names, dates, statistical numbers, locations, characteristics, descriptions, definitions, etc.

B. Exception or Negative Questions

These are fundamentally the same as the Recall Questions; but this time, the false statement serves as the correct answer.

2. Concept-oriented

These require you to understand, conclude, or judge what could be reasonably inferred from the author's views or from the evidence demonstrated in the passage.

A. Math-related Questions

This question type occasionally comes out in the RC section and calls for simple math logic, interpretation, or a quick calculation of numerical data mentioned in the passage.

B. True or False Statements

These come in two forms:

- Two Statements

Normally, a test question presents two statements, which are derived from the passage. You need to evaluate them as either both true or false, or either one of them is true or false.

- Statement and Reason

You will be presented with a cause and effect statement that requires you to judge whether the reason supports the statement or not, or both are unrelated.

C. Evaluation Questions

Some questions ask you to consider the validity, accuracy, or value of the author's ideas and/or the facts presented in the text. These heavily demand inference skills.

D. Application Questions

These questions challenge your higher cognitive skills through

generalization of the concepts presented in the passage. Use the given information to solve new problems described in the questions.

Now let's dissect and understand each question type in the following sections.

3.3.1 Recall Questions

Literal types of questions commonly appear similar to any one of the following examples:

- Term: What is the most common form of cancer?

- Statistical Number: Which of the following shows the number of times that the city was hit by an earthquake?

- Location: At which of the following countries was surgery first recognized as a legitimate medical practice?

- Synonyms: A meteor is also known as...

- Characteristics: Which of the following clinical methods characterizes the treatment used by the doctor?

- Description: The law of conservation

is stated in the passage as...

- Definition: As used in the passage, which of the following best defines "dentistry"?

Since these are primarily detail questions, most of them can be easily answered using "scan and locate" (SaL), as well as "skim for ideas" (SI) strategies.

Now let's do some exercises to ensure that you can successfully deal with these question types. Please take a piece of paper to cover the answers while you are responding to the questions. Notice that just as in the real exam, questions do not necessarily follow the chronological order of information discussed in the passage.

Read the following excerpts and promptly locate the details asked in the questions that follow.

PASSAGE 1

(1). As early as February 21, 1775, the Provincial Congress of Massachusetts appointed a committee to determine what medical supplies would be necessary should colonial troops be required to take the field. Three days later, the Congress voted to "make an inquiry where fifteen doctor's chests can be got, and on what terms"; and on March 7, it directed the committee of supplies "to make a draft in favor of Dr. Joseph Warren and Dr. Benjamin Church, for five hundred pounds, lawful money, to enable them to purchase such articles for the provincial chests of medicine as cannot be got on credit."

(2). A unique ledger of the Greenleaf apothecary shop of Boston reveals that this pharmacy on April 4, 1775, supplied at least 5 of the 15 chests of medicines. The account, in the amount of just over £247, is listed in the name of the Province of the Massachusetts Bay, and shows that £51 was paid in cash by Dr. Joseph Warren. The remaining £196 was not paid until August 10, after Warren had been killed in the Battle of Bunker Hill.

(3). The 15 medicine chests, including presumably the five supplied by Greenleaf, were distributed on April 18—three at Sudbury and two each at Concord, Groton, Mendon, Stow, Worcester, and Lancaster. No record has been found to indicate whether or not the British discovered the medical chests at Concord, but, inasmuch as the patriots were warned of the British movement, it is very likely that the chests were among the supplies that were carried off and hidden. The British destroyed as much of the remainder as they could locate.

1. What is the name of the pharmacy from which the committee purchased the medicine chests?

   Answer: _____

2. In whose account were the medical supplies listed?

   Answer: _____

3. What amount would approximately represent the price of one medicine chest?

   Answer: _____

4. Three of the medicine chests were distributed at which location?

   Answer: _____

5. The Provincial Congress of Massachusetts decided to canvass for 15 doctor's chests on which date?

   Answer: _____

PASSAGE 2

(1). The term bioinformatics was coined by Paulien Hogeweg and Ben Hesper in 1978 for the study of informatic processes in biotic systems. Its primary use since at least the late 1980s has been in genomics and genetics, particularly in those areas of genomics involving large-scale DNA sequencing. Over the past few decades rapid developments in genomic and other molecular research technologies and developments in information technologies have combined to produce a tremendous amount of information related to molecular biology.

(2). It is the name given to these mathematical and computing approaches used to glean understanding of biological processes that bioinformatics has become known as the application of computer science and information technology to the field of biology. Bioinformatics now entails the creation and advancement of databases, algorithms, computational and statistical techniques and theory to solve formal and practical problems arising from the management and analysis of biological data.

6. Bioinformatics can be defined as what?

Answer: _____

Answers:

1. Greenleaf
Strategy: Sal.; P2 S1*
(P stands for Paragraph, S stands for Sentence; the corresponding numbers point to the paragraph number and the sentence within that paragraph)

2. The Province of the Massachusetts Bay
Strategy: Sal.; P2 S2

3. 651
Strategies: Sal. and Si; P2 S2

4. Sudbury
Strategies: Sal. and Si; P3 S1

5. February 24, 1775
Strategies: Sal. and Si; P1 S2.
The Provincial Congress of Massachusetts Congress voted to "make an inquiry where fifteen doctor's chests can be got, and on what terms" three days after it appointed a committee for the medical supplies on February 21, 1775. February 21 plus 3 days makes February 24.

7. Who coined the term "bioinformatics"?

Answer: _____

8. What would characterize the main functions of bioinformatics?

Answer: _____

9. In what year did bioinformatics become useful to genomics and genetics?

Answer: _____

10. In which particular area of genomics is bioinformatics useful?

Answer: _____

Answers:

6. Bioinformatics is the application of computer science and information technology to the field of biology.
   Strategy: Sal; P2 S1

7. Paulien Hogeweg and Ben Hesper
   Strategy: Sal; P1 S1

8. Use of mathematical and computing approaches to understand biological processes
   Strategy: SI; P2 S1

9. 1980s
   Strategy: SI; P1 S2

10. large-scale DNA sequencing
    Strategy: Sal; P1 S2

3.3.2 Exception or Negative Questions

The following are some of the most common examples of this question type:

Each of the following characteristics generally pertains to modern art EXCEPT one. Which one is the EXCEPTION?

Which of the following symptoms was NOT mentioned in the passage?

Which of the following statements is false?

In these questions, using the "process of elimination" technique would be ideal in choosing the best answer out of multiple choices. There will be a number of instances when a statement would sound valid in a real world situation but is not discussed in the passage. At other times, an option would be correct but points to another closely-related concept. Therefore, you should "never lose sight of the question" as well.

PASSAGE 3

(1). Resistance to antibiotics is one of the critical complications in the treatment of infectious diseases. Enterococcal resistance to gentamicin, which is the effective antibiotic in this case, highlights the importance and the priority of the matter. Enterococci are among the most common microorganisms responsible for nosocomial infections in the hospital intensive care units and also the causative infectious agent in urinary and bile tract systems, resulting in bacteremia in infants and acute endocarditis in adults, in addition to dental and gingival infections. Therefore, isolation and identification of different enterococcal species and determination of their resistance pattern and their prevalence as well as obtaining their genetic patterns are of utmost importance. Examples of these methods include antibiogram by disk diffusion agar for determination of gentamicin resistance, evaluation of the genetic pattern utilizing DNA isolation, and observation of formed bands using electrophoresis on agarose gel 0.8% by ultraviolet. A general and comprehensive method for obtaining an ideal outcome by these methods can also be tested.

(2). Enterococci are gram-positive cocci, usually detected in feces. These bacteria grow in blood agar or BHI containing 5% blood, and are often non-hemolytic but sometimes α- or β-hemolytic. They do not produce any gases and are PYR, LAP, and bile escolin positive. They grow in 6.5% NaCl medium and can bear the 10-45°C temperature range.   The Moller Hinton medium is utilized for testing enterococcal resistance against gentamicin. In previous studies, the bacteria from diluted culture in 0.5 McFarland solution was cultured in Moller Hinton medium and the 100 µg gentamicin was placed on it and after 24 hours the resistance degree was reported by measuring the hallow around the disk. For determination of enterococcal resistance genetic pattern, the molecular and DNA derivation was used afterwards.

(3). For plasmid derivation in alkaline lysis method, plasmids are turned to deluxe rapidly. Generally, when the antibiotic concentration required for bacterial death or its growth inhibition is higher, the microorganism shows resistance to it. Plasmids are naturally circular chromosomes without any small proteins, and are seen in bacteria as well as the bacterial genome. Their genome is composed of double-stranded DNA and their replication is dependent on the host cells but independent of the bacterial genome. Most of them are replicated in bacterial reproduction cycles. Plasmids bear many genes that the bacterium usually needs their productions and for this, their high quantities are justifiable.

1.   The following are methods used for testing enterococcal resistance against

gentamicin EXCEPT one. Which is the EXCEPTION?

A. Antibiogram by Disk Diffusion Agar Test
B. The Moller Hinton medium
C. Fecal Analysis
D. Plasmid derivation in Alkaline Lysis method

2. Enterococci cause the following infections EXCEPT:

A. nosocomial infection.
B. bacteremia.
C. acute endocarditis.
D. urinary tract infection.
E. gingivitis.

3. Which is NOT a characteristic of enterococci?

A. Detected in feces
B. Do not produce any gases
C. Gram-positive cocci
D. Naturally circular chromosomes

Answers:

1. C
Strategies: SI, PoE; P1 S5, P2 S3, P3 S1 and 2

2. D
Strategies: SaL, PoE; P1 S3

3. D
Strategies: SaL, PoE; P2 S1 and S3

PASSAGE 4

(1). According to Linda Hutcheon, one of the main features that distinguishes postmodernism from modernism is the fact the it "takes the form of self-conscious, self-contradictory, self-undermining statement." One way of creating this double or contradictory stance on any statement is the use of parody: citing a convention only to make fun of it. As Hutcheon explains, "Parody—often called ironic quotation, pastiche, appropriation, or intertextuality—is usually considered central to postmodernism, both by its detractors and its defenders." Unlike Fredric Jameson, who considers such postmodern parody as a symptom of the age, one way in which we have lost our connection to the past and to effective political critique, Hutcheon argues that "through a double process of installing and ironizing, parody signals how present representations come from past ones and what ideological consequences derive from both continuity and difference."

4. Each of the following is another name for parody EXCEPT one. Which is the EXCEPTION?

A. Black Comedy
B. Ironic Quotation
C. Pastiche
D. Appropriation
E. Intertextuality

5. Which of the following is NOT a form of a postmodern statement?

    A. Self-replicating
    B. Self-conscious
    C. Self-contradictory
    D. Self-undermining

Answers:

4. A   Strategy: SaL, PoE; P1 S3

5. A   Strategy: SaL, PoE; P1 S1

3.3.3 Math-related Questions

These questions assess your comprehension of subtle mathematical relationships within a descriptive text. The following short exercises will give you an overview of how to deal with this question type.

PASSAGE 5

(1). All ordinary matter is made up of combinations of chemical elements, each with its own atomic number, indicating the number of protons in the atomic nucleus. Additionally, elements may exist in different isotopes, with each isotope of an element differing in the number of neutrons in the nucleus. A particular isotope of a particular element is called a nuclide. Some nuclides are inherently unstable. That is, at some point in time, an atom of such a nuclide will spontaneously transform into a different nuclide. This transformation may be accomplished in a number of different ways, including radioactive decay, either by emission of particles [usually electrons (beta decay), positrons or alpha particles] or by spontaneous fission, and electron capture.

(2). While the moment in time at which a particular nucleus decays is unpredictable, a collection of atoms of a radioactive nuclide decays exponentially at a rate described by a parameter known as the half-life, usually given in units of years when discussing dating techniques. After one half-life has elapsed, one half of the atoms of the nuclide in question will have decayed into a "daughter" nuclide or decay product. In many cases, the daughter nuclide itself is radioactive, resulting in a decay chain, eventually ending with the formation of a stable (nonradioactive) daughter nuclide; each step in such a chain is characterized by a distinct half-life. In these cases, usually the half-life of interest in radiometric dating is the longest one in the chain, which is the rate-limiting factor in the ultimate transformation of the radioactive nuclide into its stable daughter. Isotopic systems that have been exploited for radiometric dating have half-lives ranging from only about 10 years (e.g., tritium) to over 100 billion years.

(3). In general, the half-life of a nuclide depends solely on its nuclear properties; it is not affected by external factors such as temperature, pressure, chemical environment, or presence of a magnetic or electric field. (For some nuclides which decay by the process of electron capture, such as beryllium-7, strontium-85, and zirconium-89, the decay rate may be slightly affected by local electron density, therefore these isotopes may not be as suitable for radiometric dating.) But in general, the half-life of any nuclide is essentially a constant. Therefore, in any material containing a radioactive nuclide, the proportion of the original nuclide to its decay product(s) changes in a predictable way as the original nuclide decays over time. This predictability allows the relative abundances of related nuclides to be used as a clock to measure the time from the incorporation of the original nuclide(s) into a material to the present.

1. Based on information in the passage, how much would be left of a 5-gram radioactive nuclide parent that decays to a daughter nuclide after 3 half-lives?

Answer: _____

Answers:

1. 0.625 gram
Strategies: OA, quick calculation; P2 The passage indicates that one-half of the atoms of a parent nuclide will decay to a daughter nuclide. Thus if a parent nuclide starts out as having a value of 5 grams, it will be left with 2.5 grams after the passage of 1 half-life; 1.25 grams after the passage of two half-lives; and 0.625 after 3 half lives.

PASSAGE 6

(1). Piano music is divided by bar lines into small sections called measures. It also has numbers near the beginning of the music. These numbers are called the time signature. The time signature is related to the rhythm of the music. Each time signature contains 2 numbers: the top number tells you the number of beats or counts in each measure. The number at the bottom tells you which type of note gets the beat. A 4 at the bottom means that the QUARTER NOTE gets one beat. The 4/4 time signature is a very common time signature.

(2). The WHOLE NOTE is a white note with no stem. It receives 4 counts, or 4 beats (1-2-3-4). The HALF NOTE is a white note with a stem. It receives 2 counts (1-2). That means in the same time that you play one whole note, you could play two half notes. The QUARTER NOTE is a black note with a stem. It receives one count, or one beat. You can play 2 quarter notes in the time it takes to play a half note, or you could play 4 quarter notes in the time it takes to play a whole note.

(3). Now for the DOTTED NOTE. A dot can be slapped onto any note: whole notes, half notes, quarter notes, eighth notes, etc. Putting a dot behind a note changes the duration of the note by increasing it by half of its original value. For example: a whole note is worth 4 counts; a dotted whole note would increase the duration of the note by half of its original value (+2), so a dotted whole note would be worth 6 counts. A dotted half note would be worth 3 counts. A dotted quarter note would be worth 1 and a half counts.

2. In a 2/4 time signature, how many half notes can fit in a measure?

Answer: _____

3. Two quarter notes and one half note is equivalent to what note?

Answer: _____

4. Two dotted quarter notes would be worth how many counts?

Answer: _____

5. If an eighth note is worth half a count, how many eighth notes would it take a whole note?

Answer: _____

The "piano passage" on the actual DAT is regarded as the hardest passage, and candidates generally cringe upon encountering it. This is important to practice with - just in case.

Answers:

2. 1
Strategy: SI; P1 and P2
In the 2/4 time signature, the '2' tells us that there are 2 beats in every measure, and the '4' tells us that the quarter note gets one beat. Since a half note is worth 2 counts, this means that only 1 half note can fit a measure with 2/4 time signature.

3. Whole Note
Strategies: SaL, quick calculation; P2
One quarter note is equivalent to 1 beat, so two quarter notes equal 2 beats. One half note gets 2 beats. This means that combining two quarter notes and one half note yield 4 beats, which is equivalent to a whole note.

4. 3 quarter notes or 1 half note and 1 quarter note
Strategies: SaL, quick calculation; P3, last sentence
A dotted quarter note is worth 1 and a half counts. 1 and a half counts multiplied by 2 is 3 counts, which is either 3 quarter notes (1 beat each) or 1 half note (2 beats) and 1 quarter note (1 beat).

5. 8
Strategies: SaL, quick calculation; P2
Since a whole note is equivalent to 4 counts, this would be equivalent to 8 half counts or 8 eighth notes.

3.3.4 True or False Statements

These frequently require scanning (SaL), skimming (SI), and close attention to the surrounding details. Study the following short passages and validate the corresponding statements as any one of the following:

A. *Both statements are true.*
B. *Both statements are false.*
C. *The first statement is true. The second statement is false.*
D. *The first statement is false. The second statement is true.*

PASSAGE 7

(1). Thermodynamics is a 'phenomenal' science, in the sense that the variables of the science range over macroscopic parameters such as temperature and volume. Whether the microphysics underlying these variables are motive atoms in the void or an imponderable fluid is largely irrelevant to this science. The developers of the theory both prided themselves on this fact and at the same time worried about it. Clausius, for instance, was one of the first to speculate that heat consisted solely of the motion of particles (without an ether), for it made the equivalence of heat with mechanical work less surprising. However, as was common, he kept his "ontological" beliefs separate from his statement of the principles of thermodynamics because he didn't wish to (in his words) "taint" the latter with the speculative character of the former.

1. Macroscopic parameters refer to the philosophy underlying thermodynamics. Microphysics refers to empirical variables, such as temperature and volume.

    Answer: _____

Answer:

1. B

Strategies: SI, SaL; P1 S1 and S2

Let's have a quick refresher with the RC strategies that we used here:
SI stands for Skimming for Ideas. SaL stands for Scan and Locate. P refers to Paragraph and S to Sentence, which means that P1 S1 and S2 directs you to review Paragraph 1 Sentences 1 and 2 of the passage to find the correct answer.

PASSAGE 8

(1). Industrial noise is usually considered mainly from the point of view of environmental health and safety, rather than nuisance, as sustained exposure can cause permanent hearing damage. Traditionally, workplace noise has been a hazard linked to heavy industries such as ship-building and associated only with noise induced hearing loss (NIHL). Modern thinking in occupational safety and health identifies noise as hazardous to worker safety and health in many places of employment and by a variety of means.

(2). Noise can not only cause hearing impairment (at long-term exposures of over 85 decibels (dB), known as an exposure action value, but it also acts as a causal factor for stress and raises systolic blood pressure. Additionally, it can be a causal factor in work accidents, both by masking hazards and warning signals, and by impeding concentration. Noise also acts synergistically with other hazards to increase the risk of harm to workers. In particular, noise and dangerous substances (e.g. some solvents) that have some tendencies towards ototoxicity may give rise to rapid ear damage.

2. Occupational noise is associated only with noise induced hearing loss and heavy industries such as ship-building. Aside from hearing impairment, noise can also cause stress and elevation of systolic blood pressure.

    Answer: _____

Answer:

2. D
Strategies: SI, attention to details; P1
S2 and P2 S1

PASSAGE 9

(1). A violin consists of a body or corpus, a neck, a bridge, a soundpost, four strings, and various fittings. The fittings are the tuning pegs, tailpiece and tailgut, endpin, possibly one or more fine tuners on the tailpiece, and perhaps a chinrest, either attached directly over the tailpiece or to the left of it.

(2). The body of the violin is made of two arched plates fastened to a "garland" of ribs with animal hide glue. The rib garland includes a top block, four corner blocks (sometimes omitted in cheap mass-produced instruments,) a bottom block, and narrow strips called linings, which help solidify the curves of the ribs, and provide extra gluing surface for the plates. The ribs are what is commonly seen as the "sides" of the box. From the top or back, the body shows an "hourglass" shape formed by an upper bout and a lower bout. Two concave C-bouts between each side's corners form the waist of this figure, providing clearance for the bow.

3. Four corner blocks in the rib garland may not be found in mass-produced violins.

A chinrest is normally provided in the violin.

Answer: _____

Answer:

3. C
Strategies: SaL, attention to details; P1 S2 and P2 S2

PASSAGE 10

(1). The study of bacteria practically began with the use of the microscope. It was toward the close of the seventeenth century that the Dutch microscopist, Leeuwenhoek, working with his simple lenses, first saw the organisms which we now know under this name, with sufficient clearness to describe them. Beyond mentioning their existence, however, his observations told little or nothing. Nor can much more be said of the studies which followed during the next one hundred and fifty years. During this long period many a microscope was turned to the observation of these minute organisms, but the majority of observers were contented with simply seeing them, marveling at their minuteness, and uttering many exclamations of astonishment at the wonders of Nature.

(2). A few men of more strictly scientific natures paid some attention to these little organisms. Among them we should perhaps mention Von Gleichen, Muller, Spallanzani, and Needham. Each of these, as well as others, made some contributions to our knowledge of microscopical life, and among other organisms studied those which we now call bacteria. Speculations were even made at these early dates of the possible causal connection of these organisms with diseases, and for a little time, the medical profession was interested in the suggestion. It was impossible then, however, to obtain any evidence for the truth of this speculation, and it was abandoned as unfounded, and even forgotten completely, until revived again about the middle of the 19th century. During this century of wonder a sufficiency of exactness was, however, introduced into the study of microscopic organisms to call for the use of names, and we find Muller using the names of Monas, Proteus, Vibrio, Bacillus, and Spirillum, names which still continue in use, although commonly with a different significance from that given them by Muller. Muller did indeed make a study sufficient to recognize the several distinct types, and attempted to classify these bodies. They were not regarded as of much importance, but simply as the most minute organisms known. It was Louis Pasteur who brought bacteria to the front, and it was by his labors that these organisms were rescued from the obscurity of scientific publications and made objects of general and crowning interest.

4. Louis Pasteur was the first to recognize the existence of microscopic organisms. Muller was the first to classify the different kinds of bacteria.

Answer: _____

5. Speculations were made of the possible causal connection of microscopic organisms with diseases during the mid-18th century.
Despite little interest in the significant role of microscopic organisms to diseases, some organisms were specifically named by the mid-19th century.

Answer: _____

Answers:

4. B
Strategies: SI, attention to details; P1 S2 and P2 S2
Leeuwenhoek was the first to recognize the existence of microscopic organisms in general while Pasteur was the one who did important work specifically about the bacteria. Muller, on the other hand, classified and named the different microscopic organisms - not bacteria.

5. A
Strategies: SI; P2 S4 and S6

With questions that present a statement and a reason, careful attention to the specified details is necessary. A common decoy used is mixing up two different pieces of information from the passage, making the combination of the statement and its reason appear to be correct.

In the succeeding excerpts, let's test your acute observation of the written details. Assess the respective questions as any one of the following:

A.   *Both the statement and reason are correct and related.*
B.   *Both the statement and the reason are correct but NOT related.*
C.   *The statement is correct but the reason is NOT.*
D.   *The statement is NOT correct, but the reason is correct.*
E.   *NEITHER the statement NOR the reason is correct.*

PASSAGE 11

(1). One of the boldest and most determined of all the early explorers was Ferdinand Magellan, a young Portuguese nobleman. He felt sure that somewhere on that long coast which so many explorers had reached he would find a strait through which he would be able to pass, and which would lead into the Indian Ocean; and so Magellan formed the idea of circumnavigating the globe.

(2). He applied to the King of Portugal for aid; but as the Portuguese king was not willing to help him, he went to Spain, where his plan found favor.

(3). The Spanish king gave him a fleet of five vessels, and on September 20, 1519, he set sail for the Canary Islands. Continuing the voyage toward Sierra Leone, the vessels were becalmed, and for a period of three weeks they advanced only nine miles. Then a terrific storm arose, and the sailors, who had grumbled and found fault with everything during the entire voyage, broke into open mutiny. This mutiny Magellan quickly quelled by causing the principal offender to be arrested and put in irons.

(4). The voyage was then continued, and land was at last sighted on the Brazilian coast, near Pernambuco.

(5). The fleet then proceeded down the coast as far as Patagonia, where the weather grew so very cold that it was decided to seek winter quarters and postpone the remainder of the journey until spring. This was done, Magellan finding a sheltered spot at Port St. Julian, where plenty of fish could be obtained and where the natives were friendly.

(6). These native Patagonians Magellan described as being very tall, like giants, with long, flowing hair, and dressed scantily in skins.

(7). Great hardships had been endured by the crew. Food and water had been scarce, the storms had been severe, and suffering from cold was intense. The sailors did not believe there was any strait, and they begged Magellan to sail for home. It was useless to try to influence this determined man. Danger made him only the more firm. Magellan told them that he would not return until he had found the opening for which he was looking.

(8). Then the mutiny broke out anew. But Magellan by his prompt and decisive action put it down in twenty-four hours. One offender was killed, and two others were put in irons and left to their fate on the shore when the ships sailed away.

(9). As soon as the weather grew warmer the ships started again southward. After nearly two months of sailing, most of the time through violent storms, a narrow channel was found, in which the water was salt. This the sailors knew must be the entrance to a strait.

6. Ferdinand Magellan sought the aid of the King of Portugal because the Spanish King did not support his plan of circumnavigating the globe.

Answer: _____

7. Mutiny broke out again because the sailors found fault with everything during the entire voyage.

Answer: _____

8. Magellan formed the idea of circum-navigating the globe because he felt sure that he would find a strait through which he would be able to pass, and which would lead into the Pacific Ocean.

Answer: _____

Answers:

6. E
Strategies: Sal, attention to details; P2
The statement and the reason are reversed.

7. B
Strategies: Sl, attention to details; P3 S3, P7 and P8 S1
Details about the first mutiny was mixed up with the second mutiny.

8. C
Strategies: Sal, attention to details; P1 S2
The erroneous detail in the statement's reason is "Pacific Ocean," which should be "Indian Ocean."

PASSAGE 12

(1). Niels Henrik David Bohr was a Danish physicist who made fundamental contributions to understanding atomic structure and quantum mechanics, for which he received the Nobel Prize in Physics in 1922. Bohr mentored and collaborated with many of the top physicists of the century at his institute in Copenhagen. He was part of a team of physicists working on the Manhattan Project. Bohr married Margrethe Nørlund in 1912, and one of their sons, Aage Bohr, grew up to be an important physicist who in 1975 also received the Nobel Prize. Bohr has been described as one of the most influential scientists of the 20th century.

(2). Bohr's legacy to physics and its interpretation is a controversial one. He contributed decisively to the development of atomic and nuclear physics in many ways (especially to quantum theory from 1913 to 1925), and he is widely recognized as possessing remarkable insight into the nature of physical problems. Yet his theoretical approach and interpretive outlook sometimes have been questioned as vague, unclear, or inconsistent. Scholarship from 1970 to 2007 emphasized both the radical successes and some of the interpretive challenges of Bohr's work.

9. Bohr's legacy to physics and its interpretation is controversial because his theoretical approach and interpretive outlook have been questioned as vague, unclear, or inconsistent.

Answer: _____

10. Niels Henrik David Bohr received the Nobel Prize in Physics in 1975 for his fundamental contributions to understanding atomic structure and quantum mechanics.

Answer: _____

Answers:

9. A

Strategy: Sal.; P2 S1 and S3

10. D

Strategies: Sal., attention to details: P1 S1 and S4
The erroneous detail in the statement is the year 1975, which should 1922.

3.3.5 Evaluation Questions

Evaluation Questions mainly ask you to identify key concepts and/or facts either directly taken from the text or inferred from it. This type of question can be further subcategorized into tone, implication, and main idea questions.

- **Tone Questions**

  These entail judging the attitude or opinion of the author towards the subject.

  What is the overall tone of the passage?

  With which statement would the author of the passage agree?

- **Implication Questions**

  Based on clues and evidences in the passage, you may be asked to draw conclusions about ideas such as what would follow if the author is correct in his/her argument or what a particular discovery might lead to.

  A court jester is most likely to equate which of the following modern-day jobs?

  Which of the following is the best description of a "rocket" locomotive?

From statements in the passage, it can be inferred that the author probably is a(n)...

Which of the following sentences could best be added to the specific paragraph x?

- **Main Idea Questions**

  These test your comprehension of the theme of the article. Questions may ask you for the main idea, central idea, purpose, a possible title for the passage, and so on. You may be asked to determine which statement best expresses the author's arguments or conclusions.

  What is the main idea of the passage?

  What would be the best title for this passage?

  Which of the following sentences best fits the passage?

  Which of the following sentences is the best conclusion for the closing paragraph?

  With which statement would the author of the passage agree? (This question may border between Tone and Main Idea Questions.)

An ideal strategy for these questions would be to outline and annotate (OA). Likewise, watch out for extreme words and mean statements among the answer options.

Constant practice should help develop these strategies for the slow reader. Again, remember that the most important part of any practice is to set aside enough time to single out your mistakes, try to understand why you keep getting the wrong answers, and if you have to, modify your strategies in order to optimize your results in the actual test.

In order to get a clear gauge of your possible challenges with these question types, consider the following short passages, answer the different guide questions, and study the explanations provided.

PASSAGE 13

(1). Freud wrote several important essays on literature, which he used to explore the psyche of authors and characters, to explain narrative mysteries, and to develop new concepts in psychoanalysis (for instance, *Delusion and Dream in Jensen's Gradiva* and his influential readings of the Oedipus myth and Shakespeare's **Hamlet** in **The Interpretation of Dreams**). The criticism has been made, however, that in his and his early followers' studies "what calls for elucidation are not the artistic and literary works themselves, but rather the psychopathology and biography of the artist, writer or fictional characters." Thus many psychoanalysts among Freud's earliest adherents did not resist the temptation to psychoanalyze poets and painters sometimes to Freud's chagrin. Later analysts would conclude that "clearly one cannot psychoanalyze a writer from his text; one can only appropriate him."

1. What would be the best title for this passage?

    A. Freudian Analysis of Literary Works
    B. The Interdisciplinary Work of Freud on Classical Literature
    C. Criticisms on the Psycho-analysis of Literature
    D. Pitfalls of Psychoanalysis in Art and Literature

2. With which statement would the author of the passage agree?

    A. Freud's work has been in-fluential both in psychology and literature.
    B. One cannot always conclude about a writer's psyche based on his literary work alone.
    C. Many psychoanalysts were wrong in their findings about art and literature.
    D. Psychology and Literature can never go hand in hand.

PASSAGE 14

(1). In 1831 we have Faraday at the climax of his intellectual strength, forty years of age, stored with knowledge and full of original power. Through reading, lecturing, and experimenting, he had become thoroughly familiar with electrical science: he saw where light was needed and expansion possible. The phenomena of ordinary electric induction belonged, as it were, to the alphabet of his knowledge: he knew that under ordinary circumstances the presence of an electrified body was sufficient to excite, by induction, an unelectrified body. He knew that the wire which carried an electric current was an electrified body, and still that all attempts had failed to make it excite in other wires a state similar to its own.

(2). What was the reason of this failure? Faraday never could work from the experiments of others, however clearly described. He knew well that from every experiment issues a kind of radiation, luminous, in different degrees to different minds, and he hardly trusted himself to reason upon an experiment that he had not seen. In the autumn of 1831, he began to repeat the experiments with electric currents, which, up to that time, had produced no positive result. And here, for the sake of younger inquirers, if not for the sake of us all, it is worthwhile to dwell for a moment on a power which Faraday possessed in an extraordinary degree. He

Answers:

1. C

Strategy: OA

A title generally embodies the content, i.e., the overall idea of a specific work. Hence this question calls for understanding of the excerpt's main idea. In this paragraph, the author introduces Freud's work in analyzing various literary works then moves on to discuss various criticisms in using psychoanalysis when appraising literature and art. The keywords are "criticisms" and "psychoanalysis."

2. B

Strategies: OA (paraphrasing); extreme statements

This question requires distinguishing the author's opinion on the subject from the passage's general topic. One effective way is to watch out for structure words. A few examples are "thus," "nevertheless," "needless to say," "moreover," "however," "therefore," "on the other hand," etc. Sentences that start with these cues usually signal the author's opinion. In this example, the structure word "thus" is found in the third sentence of the paragraph: "Thus many psychoanalysts among Freud's earliest adherents did not resist the temptation to psychoanalyze poets and painters sometimes to Freud's chagrin." The author reinforces his/her view of the psychoanalysts' failure to provide faithful assessment of aesthetic works by immediately citing an example of other analysts' criticism: "Later analysts would conclude that 'clearly one cannot psychoanalyze a writer from his text; one can only appropriate him.'"

united vast strength with perfect flexibility. His momentum was that of a river, which combines weight and directness with the ability to yield to the flexures of its bed. The intentness of his vision in any direction did not apparently diminish his power of perception in other directions; and when he attacked a subject, expecting results, he had the faculty of keeping his mind alert, so that results different from those which he expected should not escape him through pre-occupation.

3. Which of the following sentences is the best conclusion for the closing paragraph?

   A. Faraday finally sought the advice of other scientists working on a similar experiment.

   B. Unfortunately, Faraday had to abandon his work.

   C. Luckily, Faraday found the missing element that would make his experiment successful.

   D. And so, Faraday persevered in conducting his experiments with electric currents.

4. Which of the following sentences best fits the passage?

   A. Faraday was a genius in electrical science.

   B. Faraday's failure was directly related to his refusal to colla-

borate with other scientists.

   C. Faraday was a man of great intellectual insights and determination.

   D. Faraday was a stubborn scientist.

Answers:

3. D

Strategy: QA or SI

The overall tone of the passage is that of optimism and admiration for Faraday's perseverance and intellectual independence. A and B are exact opposites of the statements in P2 S2 to S3 and P2 S7 respectively. C does not have enough clue or clear evidence as basis. D matches the characteristics described by the author about Faraday.

4. C

Strategy: QA or SI

This is a main idea question, which means that the best choice should be the statement that most represents the central point of the passage. Paragraph 1 discusses the extent of Faraday's knowledge especially about electrical science. Paragraph 2 illustrates Faraday's persistence despite failures in his experiments. Therefore, the most encompassing idea about the passage is that of Option C. A and B, although true, are only mentioned in specific parts of Paragraph 1 and Paragraph 2 respectively. D misinterprets the author's characterization of Faraday.

PASSAGE 15

(1). This project was inspired by a number of visits I made to various science and engineering museums in order to investigate the design of small electronic consumer devices. The research trips were unsuccessful, but only in the sense that my original expectations had not been met. I found that the objects on display in most cases looked exactly like the final product that would then be presented to the market. I had expected to see unfinished hotchpotches of machines, exposed working components and a cacophony of tangled cables. I was also hoping for a look beyond, or behind, the scenes of the design process and into a space manufacturers might ordinarily keep from public view. Instead, the objects that I came across were merely empty shells, made only to demonstrate the aesthetic of the product's design.

5. What is the overall tone of the passage?

   A. Disgust
   B. Disappointment
   C. Businesslike
   D. Curious

6. From statements in the passage, it can be inferred that the author probably is a(n):

   A. art critic.
   B. tourist.
   C. auctioneer.
   D. engineer.

Answers:

5. B
Strategy: SI: P1 S2 and S6

6. A
Strategy: SI: P1 S1 and last sentence
In both sentences, the author referred to "design" and "aesthetic of the product's design." A tourist would not be too critical; an auctioneer would have mentioned something about a bid; and, an engineer would not keep considering the "aesthetics of a product's design."

DAT-Prep.com
GOLD STANDARD DAT RC

3.3.6 Application Questions

These are questions involving concepts that were introduced in the passage and how they would apply to general or real world situations. Usually, a situation or function is given, and you will be made to identify which particular theory, process, or instrument would best fit the description or offer a solution. You should use the information presented in the passage to solve new problems described in the questions; reevaluate the passage based on new facts associated with the questions.

Possible effective strategies could include "scan and locate" (SaL), "skim for ideas" (SI), "outline and annotate" (OA) or sketch the described apparatus or process in order to concretize the concepts.

PASSAGE 16

(1). There still exists among ourselves an activity, which on the technical plane gives us quite a good understanding of what a science we prefer to call 'prior' rather than 'primitive,' could have been on the plane of speculation. This is what is commonly called 'bricolage' in French. In its old sense the verb 'bricoler' applied to ball games and billiards, to hunting, shooting and riding. It was however always used with reference to some extraneous movement: a ball rebounding, a dog straying or a horse swerving from its direct course to avoid an obstacle. And in our own time the 'bricoleur' is still someone who works with his hands and uses devious means compared to those of a craftsman.

(2). The 'bricoleur' is adept at performing a large number of diverse tasks; but, unlike the engineer, he does not subordinate each of them to the availability of raw materials and tools conceived and procured for the purpose of the project. His universe of instruments is closed and the rules of his game are always to make do with 'whatever is at hand', that is to say with a set of tools and materials which is always finite and is also heterogeneous because what it contains bears no relation to the current project, or indeed to any particular project, but is the contingent result of all the occasions there have been to renew or enrich the stock or to maintain it with the remains of previous constructions or destructions.

(3). The set of the bricoleur's means cannot therefore be defined in terms of a project (which would presuppose besides, that, as in the case of the engineer, there were, at least in theory, as many sets of tools and materials or 'instrumental sets', as there are different kinds of projects). It is to be defined only by its potential use or, putting this another way and in the language of the 'bricoleur' himself, because the elements are collected or retained on

RC-62   CHAPTER 3: DAT READING COMPREHENSION STRATEGIES

the principle that 'they may always come in handy'. Such elements are specialized up to a point, sufficiently for the 'bricoleur' not to need the equipment and knowledge of all trades and professions, but not enough for each of them to have only one definite and determinate use. They each represent a set of actual and possible relations; they are 'operators' but they can be used for any operations of the same type.

1. Which of the following constructions below would NOT be an example of "bricolage"?

   A. Scrapbooking
   B. Surrealistic Poetry
   C. Junk Art
   D. A Land Survey
   E. Decorative Food Servings

2. Which activity would NOT be an illustration of "bricolage"?

   A. Stage sets made up of scrap metal for a theatrical performance
   B. A birdhouse constructed from toothpicks and various wood scraps
   C. A well-designed deck with pre-cut lumber
   D. A quilt sewn together with various leftover fabrics
   E. A maze constructed from the various hedges and shrubs in the garden

3. The Digital Era and Computer Apps have given bricolage a refreshing outlook due to advanced manipulation of popular media. Which entries BEST represent a type of digital "bricolage"?

   A. Using digital audio loops (cut and paste) for recording mixes and remixes
   B. GPS used in other contexts such as cruise ships, restaurants, etc.
   C. Photoshopped pictures, which distort the original to something humorous
   D. Constructing a website

Answers:

1. D
   Strategy: SI; P1 last sentence, P2 S1, P3 S1
   Scrapbooking, surrealistic poetry, junk art, and decorative food servings all entail "working with hands" and using "devious means." On the other hand, land surveying would require using instruments, calculations and some engineering background.

2. C
   Strategy: SaL or OA; P1 and P2
   Descriptions in the passage suggest that bricolage would involve making do with "whatever is at hand." Only a well-designed deck with lumber cut to a specific shape or size would not fit this description.

3. A
   Strategy: SaL; P2 last sentence
   "His universe of instruments is closed and the rules of his game are always to make do with 'whatever is at hand', that is to say with a set of tools and materials which is always finite and is also heterogeneous because what it contains bears no relation to the current project, or indeed to any particular project, but is the contingent result of all the occasions there have been to renew or enrich the stock or to maintain it with the remains of previous constructions or destructions."

Chapter Checklist

☐ Sign up or access your free online account at www.dat-prep.com to join the forum to discuss any content from this chapter or any practice questions in this Masters Series book.

☐ Identify the strategies and techniques that worked best for you. Commit to either using those strategies and techniques for the upcoming GS mini tests, or at least using different strategies in different tests to objectively confirm which ones work best for you.

☐ Complete a maximum of 1 page of notes using symbols/abbreviations to represent the entire chapter. These are your Gold Notes.

☐ Consider your options based on your optimal way of learning:

☐ Create your own, tangible study cards or try the free app: Anki.

☐ Record your voice reading your Gold Notes onto your smartphone (MP3s) and listen during exercise, transportation, etc. (*see RC 2.5 as an example*).

☐ Consider reading at least 1 source material every day (*see RC 2.2.1*). Note down the main idea or ideas of the piece on your scratch paper or noteboard. Determine or surmise the author's sentiment or purpose for writing the material.

☐ Schedule your full-length DAT practice tests: ADA and/or GS exams and/or other free or paid third-party resources. Schedule one full day to complete a practice test and 1-2 days for a thorough assessment of answers and explanations while adding to your abbreviated Gold Notes.

☐ Schedule and/or evaluate stress reduction techniques such as regular exercise (sports), yoga, meditation and/or mindfulness exercises (*see* YouTube for suggestions).

GOLD STANDARD DAT
RC MINI TESTS (4)

4.1 Reading Comprehension (RC) Mini Tests with Answer Key, Explanations and Strategies

Now that we have outlined the structure of the DAT Reading Comprehension section, the types of questions, and most importantly, the approach and strategies that will help you excel, you can proceed to test yourself with our GS RC mini tests.

As described earlier, the DAT RC is comprised of three passages. A mini test presents only one passage at a time. The objective is to get you started in applying the techniques discussed in sections 3.1 to 3.3, and allow you to assess your current level of competence. We strongly suggest that you ALWAYS time yourself for every practice test. Otherwise, you would be eliminating one of the major components of your preparation making it more difficult to get a top DAT RC score.

At the end of each mini test, you should work through the answers and explanations. The answer key specifies the **Question Type** and the **Strategies** that are appropriate for the question. Keep notes of your wrong answers and then go back to the specific section(s) in this chapter, reviewing and analyzing how you can still improve on your next attempts. Only when you feel ready, you can try to get an initial run of the whole RC exam by taking the full-length GS RC Practice Test at the end of the Reading Comprehension chapters. As you progress with your review, you should also consider full-length practice tests (i.e. NS, PAT, RC and QR in one sitting) including those from the ADA, Gold Standard and/or other third party resources.

Before you proceed, let's reiterate some important abbreviations and references in our answer keys:

OA	Outline and Annotate	Discussed in Section 3.3
SaL	Scan and Locate	Discussed in Section 3.3
SI	Skim for Ideas	Discussed in Section 3.3
PoE	Process of Elimination	Discussed in Section 3.2
Attention to details		Discussed in Section 3.2
Never lose sight of the question		Discussed in Section 3.2
P	Paragraph	P1 would mean Paragraph 1 and so forth
S	Sentence	S1 would mean Sentence 1 and so forth

*A note on "Recall Questions": Most recall questions do not need detailed explanations and only require you to re-read a specific paragraph and sentence. Hence only the paragraph and sentence numbers are provided in the answer key explanations of some of these questions.

From this point, advance to the next pages ONLY when you are ready. Please give each attempt your best shot. Good luck!

RC Mini Test 1

The following is a sample mini test which is comparable to the level of difficulty required for the Reading Comprehension Test of the DAT. Please note that this sample would roughly be 1/3 of the actual Reading Comprehension Test portion of the DAT.

You have 20 minutes to complete this portion of the DAT Mini Test; the actual test is 60 minutes. Please time yourself accordingly.

> BEGIN ONLY WHEN YOUR TIMER IS READY.

Passage 1

NASA Science Balloons

(1). Balloons may seem like an old-fashioned technology to most of the public, but they are very much alive and well. Weather balloons have been commonplace for decades, and the military still makes considerable use of them. The public is very familiar with hot-air sport ballooning, as well as with the exciting record-breaking flights across continents and oceans, using very high-tech balloon technologies. While the "great age" of manned balloon flights into the stratosphere is history, balloons continue to be important tools for scientific research. Unmanned stratospheric balloons are used for astronomy and climate studies, and balloons are also potentially an important tool for exploring other planets.

(2). The US National Science Foundation set up a scientific balloon program in 1961, originally based in Boulder, Colorado. In 1963, the balloon program was moved to Palestine, Texas, halfway between Dallas and Houston, since at the time the area was largely unpopulated and balloon payloads falling out of the sky were unlikely to land on a house. The US National Aeronautics & Space Administration (NASA) picked up the balloon program in 1982. The Palestine operation is now designated the "Columbia Scientific Balloon Facility (CSBF)" – the name having been changed from the "National Scientific Balloon Facility" in 2005 in honor of the crew of the space shuttle Columbia, which burned up on reentry in 2003.

(3). The CSBF is directed by the Physical

Sciences Laboratory of New Mexico State University at Las Cruces. However, population growth near Palestine has forced the CSBF to perform more launches at remote sites. Launches are regularly performed at Fort Sumner, New Mexico; Lynn Lake, Manitoba, Canada; McMurdo Station, Antarctica; Fairbanks, Alaska; and Alice Springs, Australia. Special launches have also been performed from a number of other locales. The CSBF has performed over 2,000 balloon flights since its inception. At its peak, in the 1970s, the CSBF was performing up to 80 missions a year, but the organization's launch rate is now much lower, a few dozen missions a year. Partly this is because the feasible missions have mostly been done, but it is also due to funding limitations. However, the CSBF is not in danger of extinction, since researchers know that it is much easier, quicker, and cheaper to use a balloon than a spacecraft to fly a payload into near-space conditions. The fact that balloon payloads, unlike satellite payloads, are usually recovered intact for re-use is another plus.

(4). The modern "zero-pressure balloon" vehicle used by the CSBF is generally similar to the SKYHOOK balloons originally invented by Otto Winzen. It is made from special polyethylene film, typically 0.8 mil thick, fabricated from longitudinal panels sealed with tapes. A scientific balloon typically has a volume of 1.08 million cubic meters (38 million cubic feet) and can carry 1,700 kilograms (3,750 pounds) of suspended load to 39 kilometers (128,000 feet). At this altitude, the scientific payload is above 99.7% of the atmosphere's mass. The "flight train" consists of the balloon and a scientific instrument package hitched to the balloon through a parachute pack. A NASA zero-pressure science balloon is inflated through the traditional roller system, with enough lifting gas provided for 10% lift over the load and balloon mass, and the gas expanding as the balloon rises.

(5). Data from the payload and balloon are telemetered directly to ground stations or through satellite links. Occasionally they are also recorded on board via film, magnetic tape, or solid-state digital storage media. Radio commands are used for instrument and balloon control. Balloon position is obtained by direct visual tracking, airplane tracking, or use of Global Position System (GPS) navigation receivers. The flight ends when the parachute and payload are separated via radio command, usually from a tracking aircraft. During separation, the balloon is destroyed by tearing open a set of rip panels, permitting the payload to parachute to the ground. With recent improvements in design, materials, and quality control, the large zero-pressure balloon has become an extremely reliable vehicle, with very high mission success rates. One drawback, however, is its limited mission endurance. While long-standing studies on cosmic rays, atmospheric circulation, and weather continue, much recent effort has been devoted to the atmospheric chemistry, and to astronomy at wavelengths – such as the infrared, ultraviolet, and X-ray bands – that are blocked by the atmosphere.

(6). An alternative approach, the "constant volume" or "superpressure" balloon, features a relatively unyielding plastic envelope filled at relatively high pressure, ensuring retention of a constant volume. A superpressure balloon does not need ballast, or at least not as much as a zero-pressure balloon, and can float at high altitudes for many months. The CSBF is now working on a superpressure "Ultra-Long Duration Balloon (ULDB)" that can stay at altitude for several months, orbiting the Earth several times. Raven Industries conducted a flight of a prototype ULDB in October 1999, but the balloon ruptured when it reached altitude. A second prototype, a tenth the size of a full-scale ULDB, was launched in June 2000 and was a success, remaining aloft for 27 hours. The full-scale ULDB design features an envelope with an inflated diameter of 59 meters (193 feet) and a height of 35 meters (115 feet). It is intended to remain aloft with 900 kilograms (a ton) of payload at altitudes of 35 kilometers (115,000 feet) for up to 100 days. The first full-scale ULDB test flight took place in late February 2001 from an Alice Springs, Australia launch site, but sprung a leak and was destroyed a few hours after launch. Subsequent launches took place roughly once a year, with mixed results. NASA still plans to begin operational ULDB launches in 2010.

(7). The superpressure balloon concept is not entirely new, going back at least to the US Air Force's "Global Horizontal Sounding Technique (GHOST)" balloon program, with eighty-eight GHOST balloons about 3 meters (10 feet) in diameter released over a period of ten years beginning in 1966. They all carried a small payload, the primary goal of the mission being to simply track the balloons to map high-altitude winds. In 1966, a GHOST balloon was the first balloon to circle the Earth, taking ten days to make the journey. Some of the GHOST balloons were said to have remained aloft for a year. Later in the program, they relayed their data through satellites. This project provided new results on the seasonal variations of global air currents.

(8). Balloons have proven very useful for scientific research on Earth; there are those who believe they are potentially very useful for exploring other planets as well. Robot "rovers" have been sent to the Moon and Mars since the 1960s, but such machines tend to be expensive and have limited range, and due to the long communications time-lag over interplanetary distances, they have to be smart enough to navigate without running into obstacles or falling off cliffs. If a planet has an atmosphere, however, a balloon would have many advantages over a rover. A robot balloon, or "aerobot", would be much cheaper and lighter than a rover, with the light weight reducing booster launch costs. An aerobot could cover a great deal of ground, and its view from a height would give them the ability to examine wide swathes of terrain with far more detail than would be obtained by an orbiting satellite. For exploratory missions, the aerobot's relative lack of directional control would not be a big concern, since there would be generally no need to direct it to a specific location. While the French were working on planetary aerobots, NASA's Jet Propulsion Laboratory (JPL) had become interested in the idea as well, with a JPL team performing several balloon flights in the Earth's atmosphere during the 1990s to validate technology. The JPL team envisioned a simple "Mars weather balloon" to validate the technology operationally; to be followed by a large superpressure balloon flight; and finally a solar-powered Mars blimp. NASA hasn't committed to an aerobot mission yet, but the agency has collaborated with the Centre National d'Études Spatiales (CNES) on the development of a series of low-cost "Scout" missions to Mars, and a Mars aerobot is on the list of options. A company named Global Aerospace Corporation performed an investigation of a Mars aerobot for NASA, with the aerobot envisioned as carrying both a science gondola and a set of small drop probes that could be released to provide detailed inspection of a number of sites.

- Adapted from "NASA Science Balloons" (http://www.vectorsite.net/avbloon_5.html#m1) Thanks to Greg Goebel.

1. Of the regular balloon launch sites, which of the following is NOT listed in the article?

   A. Fort Sumner
   B. Lynn Lake
   C. Columbia
   D. Alice Springs
   E. Fairbanks

2. The US National Science Foundation set up a scientific balloon program in 1961. NASA set up a similar program in 1963.

   A. Both statements are true.
   B. Both statements are false.
   C. The first sentence is true. The second sentence is false.
   D. The first sentence is false. The second sentence is true.
   E. The passage does not contain enough information to make a judgment.

3. Of the balloons discussed in the passage, which is NOT mentioned? Which is the EXCEPTION?

   A. Zero-pressure balloons
   B. Hot air balloons
   C. Superpressure balloons
   D. Weather balloons
   E. Anisotropic balloons

4. Which balloon provided new results on the seasonal variations of global air currents?

   A. Ultra-Long Duration balloon
   B. GHOST balloons
   C. Anisotropic balloons
   D. Zero-pressure balloons
   E. Aerobot balloons

5. Which of the following is NOT true about the modern zero-pressure balloons used by CSBF?

A. It can remain aloft for 27 hours.
B. It has a typical volume of 1.08 million cubic meters.
C. It is typically 0.8 mil thick, made of special polyethylene film.
D. It can typically carry 3750 pounds of suspended load.
E. None of the above

6. Which of the following acronyms is NOT correct?

A. JPL - Jet Propulsion Laboratory
B. GHOST - Global Horizontal Sounding Technique
C. ULDB - Ultra-Long Duration Balloon
D. CSBF - Columbia Super Balloon Facility
E. NASA - National Aeronautics & Space Administration

7. In the 1970s, CSBF was performing up to:

A. 80 missions a year.
B. 88 missions a year.
C. 70 missions a year.
D. 800 missions a year.
E. 90 missions a year.

8. The space shuttle Columbia burned up on reentry in which of the following years?

A. 2005
B. 1982
C. 1962
D. 2003
E. 2000

9. Based on statements in the passage, it can be inferred that a "payload" is:

A. a tracking device.
B. a communication device.
C. a data collection device.
D. the total weight of all of the balloons.
E. total balloon contents.

10. Each of the following statements is true concerning the latest ULDBs EXCEPT one. Which one is the EXCEPTION?

A. It has an inflated diameter of 193 feet.
B. It has an inflated height of 115 feet.
C. It can carry up to a ton of payload.
D. It can carry a ton of payload for 100 days.
E. It can carry a ton of payload at altitudes over 200,000 feet.

11. Which of the following was the first balloon to circle the Earth?

A. ULDB
B. Aerobot
C. GHOST
D. SKYHOOK
E. Solar-powered blimp

12. The primary goal of a GHOST balloon was:

A. to interlink with satellites.
B. to map high-altitude winds.
C. to understand atmospheric chemistry.
D. to study cosmic rays.
E. to provide geographical surveillance.

13. Balloon payloads are usually recovered intact.

Satellite payloads, on the other hand, are much cheaper to use.

A. Both statements are true.
B. Both statements are false.
C. The first statement is true, the second statement is false.
D. The first statement is false, the second statement is true.

14. The first full-scale ULDB test flight took place in late February 2001 from which of the following locations?

A. Fort Sumner
B. Lynn Lakes
C. Fairbanks
D. Alice Springs
E. Palestine

15. From the following list of popular narratives, which would be the most relevant to the article?

A. Moby Dick
B. Hamlet
C. Ulysses
D. 20,000 Leagues Under the Sea
E. Around the World in 80 days

16. Each of the following would be an advantage of a Mars Aerobot over a Mars Rover EXCEPT one. Which one is the EXCEPTION?

A. Cost
B. Range
C. Predictability of direction
D. Weight
E. Details of view

17. The improved large zero-pressure balloon has very low mission success rates.
Yet, this version has very high mission
endurance.

A. Both statements are true.

B. Both statements are false.

C. The first statement is true, while
the second statement is false.

D. The first statement is false, while
the second statement is true.

> If time remains, you may review your
> work. If your allotted time (20 minutes)
> is complete, please proceed to the
> Answer Key.

RC Mini Test 1 Answer Key

1. C	7. A	13. C
2. C	8. D	14. D
3. E	9. C	15. E
4. B	10. E	16. C
5. A	11. C	17. B
6. D	12. B	

RC Mini Test 1 Explanations and Strategies

1. Question Type: *Exception/Negative Question*
Strategies: *SaL, PoE; P3 S3, P2 last sentence*

(A) Fort Sumner, (B) Lynn Lake, (D) Alice Springs and (E) Fairbanks are all mentioned in Paragraph 3. On the other hand, Columbia was the name of the space shuttle that burned up in 2003 as indicated in the last sentence of Paragraph 2.

2. Question Type: *True False Statement (Two Statements)*
Strategies: *SaL, attention to details; P2 S1 to S3*

The third sentence of Paragraph 2 states that NASA picked up the balloon program in 1982, not 1963.

3. Question Type: *Exception/Negative Question*
Strategies: *SaL, PoE*

Paragraph 4 discusses (A) zero-pressure balloons and Paragraph 6 (C) superpressure balloons. (D) Weather balloons is mentioned in P1 S2 and (B) hot air balloons in P1 S3. Only (E) anisotropic balloons are not mentioned anywhere in the passage.

4. Question Type: *Recall*
Strategy: *SaL; P7 last sentence*

5. Question Type: *Exception/Negative Question*
Strategies: *SaL, PoE, attention to details*

The modern zero-pressure balloons are discussed in Paragraph 4, specifically Statement B in S3, Statement C in S2, and Statement

D in S3. On the other hand, Statement A is mixed up with the information in P6 S5, which supposedly pertains to the ULDB superpressure balloon – not the zero-pressure balloons used by CSBF.

6. Question Type: *Exception/Negative Question*
    Strategies: *SaL, PoE, attention to details*

    JPL is mentioned in P8 S7, GHOST in P7 S1, ULDB in P6 S3, and NASA in P2 S3. CSBF is indeed mentioned in P2 S4 but as Columbia Scientific Balloon Facility – not Columbia Super Balloon Facility.

7. Question Type: *Recall*
    Strategy: *SaL; P3 S6*

8. Question Type: *Recall*
    Strategy: *SaL; P2 last sentence*

9. Question Type: *Evaluation Question*
    Strategies: *SI, attention to details; P5 S1 to S5*

    Several contextual cue words in the first 5 sentences of Paragraph 5 hint that a payload functions as a data collection device: "Data from the payload and balloon are telemetered," "recorded on board via film, magnetic tape, or solid-state digital storage media," "direct visual tracking, airplane tracking, or use of Global Position System (GPS) navigation receivers."

10. Question Type: *Exception/Negative Question*
    Strategies: *SaL, PoE; P6*

    Each answer choice is mentioned in the following specific sentences in Paragraph 6: A and B in S6; C and D in S7. Only the data in E cannot be found in the paragraph or anywhere in the passage.

11. Question Type: *Recall*
    Strategies: *SaL; P7 S3*

12. Question Type: *Recall*
    Strategy: *SaL; P7 S2*

13. Question Type: *True False Statement (Two Statements)*
    Strategies: *SaL, PoE, attention to details; P3 S8 and last sentence*

    The first statement is true as indicated in P3 last sentence. However, the second statement is false: balloon payloads - NOT satellite payloads - are cheaper.

14. Question Type: *Recall*
    Strategy: *SaL; P6 S7*

15. Question Type: *Evaluation Question (Main Idea)*
    Strategies: *SI, prior knowledge*

    This question can be easily answered with simple inference and familiarity with the titles presented in the different choices. Understanding that the passage is about air balloons or balloon flights, the narrative that has this same theme should match as the correct answer.

16. Question Type: *Exception/Negative Question*
Strategies: *SI, PoE, attention to details; P8 S4 to S6*

Answering this question may require more attention to details because the answer choices are paraphrased from lines in the passage. (A) Cost would equate "aerobot would be much cheaper"; (B) Range would be "could cover a great deal of ground"; (C) Predictability of direction would be "lack of directional control," which is not considered as an aerobot's advantage over a rover – therefore,

the correct answer; (D) weight is "lighter than a rover"; and (E) Details of view is "the ability to examine wide swathes of terrain with far more detail."

17. Question Type: *True False Statement (Two statements)*
Strategies: *SaL, attention to details; P5 S7 and S8*

The information in the two statements are reversed.

Would you like to discuss any of the answers
or strategies in this section?
Go to www.dat-prep.com/forum to share and learn.

RC Mini Test 2

The following is a sample mini test which is comparable to the level of difficulty required for the Reading Comprehension Test of the DAT. Please note that this sample would roughly be 1/3 of the actual Reading Comprehension Test portion of the DAT.

You have 20 minutes to complete this portion of the DAT Mini Test; the actual test is 60 minutes. Please time yourself accordingly.

BEGIN ONLY WHEN YOUR TIMER IS READY.

Passage 2

Symbiosis

(1). Symbiosis (from Ancient Greek sýn "with" and bíōsis "living") is a close and often long-term interaction between different biological species. In 1877, Bennett used the word symbiosis (which previously had been used for people living together in community) to describe the mutualistic relationship in lichens. In 1879, the German mycologist Heinrich Anton de Bary defined it as "the living together of unlike organisms." The definition of symbiosis is controversial among scientists. Some believe symbiosis should only refer to persistent mutualisms, while others believe it should apply to all types of persistent biological interactions (i.e., mutualistic, commensalistic, or parasitic).

(2). Some symbiotic relationships are obligate, meaning that both symbionts entirely depend on each other for survival. For example, many lichens consist of fungal and photosynthetic symbionts that cannot live on their own. Others are facultative, meaning that they can but do not have to live with the other organism. Symbiotic relationships include those associations in which one organism lives on another (ectosymbiosis, such as mistletoe), or where one partner lives inside the other (endosymbiosis, such as lactobacilli and other bacteria in humans or zooxanthellae in corals).

(3). Endosymbiosis is any symbiotic relationship in which one symbiont lives within the tissues of the other, either in the intracellular or extracellular space. Examples are rhizobia, nitrogen-fixing bacteria that live in root nodules on legume roots; actinomycete nitrogen-fixing bacteria called Frankia, which live in alder tree root nodules; single-celled algae inside reef-building corals; and bacterial endosymbionts that provide essential nutrients to about 10%–15% of insects. Ectosymbiosis, also referred to as exosymbiosis, is any symbiotic relationship in which the symbiont lives on the body surface of the host, including the inner surface of the digestive tract or the ducts of exocrine glands. Examples of this include ectoparasites such as lice, commensal ectosymbionts such as the barnacles that attach themselves to the jaw of baleen whales, and mutualist ectosymbionts such as cleaner fish.

(4). Mutualism is any relationship between individuals of different species where both individuals derive a benefit. Generally, only lifelong interactions involving close physical and biochemical contact can properly be considered symbiotic. Mutualistic relationships may be either obligate for both species, obligate for one but facultative for the other, or facultative for both. Many biologists restrict the definition of symbiosis to close mutualist relationships. A large percentage of herbivores have mutualistic gut fauna that help them digest plant matter, which is more difficult to digest than animal prey. Coral reefs are the result of mutualisms between coral organisms and various types of algae that live inside them. Most land plants and land ecosystems rely on mutualisms between the plants, which fix carbon from the air, and mycorrhizal fungi, which help in extracting minerals from the ground.

(5). An example of mutual symbiosis is the relationship between the ocellaris clownfish that dwell among the tentacles of Ritteri sea anemones. The territorial fish protects the anemone from anemone-eating fish, and in turn the stinging tentacles of the anemone protect the clownfish from its predators. A special mucus on the clownfish protects it from the stinging tentacles. Another example is the goby fish, which sometimes lives together with a shrimp. The shrimp digs and cleans up a burrow in the sand in which both the shrimp and the goby fish live. The shrimp is almost blind, leaving it vulnerable to predators when above ground. In case of danger the goby fish touches the shrimp with its tail to warn it. When that happens, both the shrimp and goby fish quickly retract into the burrow.

(6). One of the most spectacular examples of obligate mutualism is between the siboglinid tube worms and symbiotic bacteria that live at hydrothermal vents and cold seeps. The worm has no digestive tract and is wholly reliant on its internal symbionts for nutrition. The bacteria oxidize either hydrogen sulfide or methane, which the host supplies to them. These worms were discovered in the late 1980s at the hydrothermal vents near the Galapagos Islands and have since been found at deep-sea hydrothermal vents and cold seeps in all of the world's oceans. There are also many types of tropical and sub-tropical ants that have evolved very complex relationships with certain tree species.

(7). Commensalism describes a relationship between two living organisms where one benefits and the other is not significantly harmed or helped. It is derived from the English word commensal, used for human social interaction. The word derives from the medieval Latin word, formed from "com" and "mensa," meaning "sharing a table." Commensal relationships may involve one organism using another for transportation (phoresy) or for housing (inquilinism), or it may also involve one organism using something that another created after its death (metabiosis). Examples of metabiosis are maggots, which feast and develop on corpses, and hermit crabs using gastropod shells to protect their bodies.

(8). A parasitic relationship is one in which one member of the association benefits while the other is harmed. Parasitic symbioses take many forms, from endoparasites that live within the host's body to ectoparasites that live on its surface. In addition, parasites may be necrotrophic, which is to say they kill their host, or biotrophic, meaning they rely on their host's surviving. Biotrophic parasitism is an extremely successful mode of life. Depending on the definition used, as many as half of all animals have at least one parasitic phase in their life cycles, and it is also frequent in plants and fungi. Moreover, almost all free-living animals are host to one or more parasite taxa. An example of a biotrophic relationship would be a tick feeding on the blood of its host.

(9). Amensalism is the type of symbiotic relationship that exists where one species is inhibited or completely obliterated and one is unaffected. This type of symbiosis is relatively uncommon in rudimentary reference texts, but is omnipresent in the natural world. An example is a sapling growing under the shadow of a mature tree. The mature tree can begin to rob the sapling of necessary sunlight and, if the mature tree is very large, it can take up rainwater and deplete soil nutrients. Throughout the process the mature tree is unaffected. Indeed, if the sapling dies, the mature tree gains nutrients from the decaying sapling. Note that these nutrients become available because of the sapling's decomposition, rather than from the living sapling, which would be a case of parasitism.

(10). While historically, symbiosis has received less attention than other interactions such as predation or competition, it is increasingly recognized as an important selective force behind evolution, with many species having a long history of interdependent co-evolution. In fact, the evolution of all eukaryotes (plants, animals, fungi, and protists) is believed under the endosymbiotic theory to have resulted from a symbiosis between various sorts of bacteria. Up to 80% of vascular plants worldwide form symbiotic relationships with fungi, for example, in arbuscular mycorrhiza.

(11). The biologist Lynn Margulis, famous for her work on endosymbiosis, contends that symbiosis is a major driving force behind evolution. She considers Darwin's notion of evolution, driven by competition, to be incomplete and claims that evolution is strongly based on co-operation, interaction, and mutual dependence among organisms. According to Margulis and Dorion Sagan, "Life did not take over the globe by combat, but by networking."

(12). Symbiosis played a major role in the co-evolution of flowering plants and the animals that pollinate them. Many plants that are pollinated by insects, bats, or birds have highly specialized flowers modified to promote pollination by a specific pollinator that is also correspondingly adapted. The first flowering plants in the fossil record had relatively simple flowers. Adaptive speciation quickly gave rise to many diverse groups of plants, and, at the same time, corresponding speciation occurred in certain insect groups. Some groups of plants developed nectar and large sticky pollen, while insects evolved more specialized morphologies to access and collect these rich food sources. In some taxa of plants and insects the relationship has become dependent, where the plant species can only be pollinated by one species of insect.

1. Understory vegetation grows beneath the breeding colonies of herons. As the heron's population becomes dense, the trees on which they build their nests eventually die down due to the bird's heavy toxic excrements. The herons may suffer from the loss of their nesting trees, but they do not necessarily get hurt or benefit from the damaged vegetation. This type of symbiotic relationship is described to be:

   A. commensalism.
   B. parasitism.
   C. amensalism.
   D. ectosymbiosis.

2. In the example of mutual symbiosis between the shrimp and the goby fish, what is the primary benefit of their relationship?

   A. Protection
   B. Shelter
   C. Nutrition
   D. Transportation
   E. Propagation

3.   Each of the following are considered mutually beneficial symbionts EXCEPT one.   Which one is the EXCEPTION?

   A.   Rhizobia
   B.   Bacterial endosymbionts
   C.   Lice
   D.   Frankia
   E.   Lactobacilli

4.   Which of the following best describes symbiosis?

   A.   The ability of unlike organisms to live together
   B.   Close relationship between two different species
   C.   Lifelong close physical and biochemical contact of different species
   D.   Persistent biological interactions in a community of diverse species
   E.   Long-term mutually beneficial relationships of different biological species

5.   Termites can chew and ingest wood, but they rely on their intestinal flagellates trichonympha to break down their food for them and chemically digest cellulose into sugars. The termite, in turn, provides food, shelter and constant internal environment to the trichonympha. Both cannot survive in the absence of the other. This type of relationship is an example of:

   A.   inquilinism.
   B.   necrotrophic parasitism.
   C.   biotrophic parasitism.
   D.   obligate mutualism.
   E.   facultative mutualism.

6.   Most orchids are plants that depend on their hosts for physical support and not nutrition. To which of the following symbiotic interaction would orchids belong?

   A.   Ectoparasitism
   B.   Biotrophic parasitism
   C.   Facultative mutualism
   D.   Metabiosis
   E.   Inquilinism

7. Historically, symbiosis has received less attention than predation and competition.

   Yet, it is believed as an important selective force behind the evolution of eukaryotes.

   A. Both statements are true.
   B. Both statements are false.
   C. The first sentence is true while the second sentence is false.
   D. The first sentence is false while the second sentence is true.

8. Ectosymbiosis is the same as:

   A. ectoparasitism.
   B. endosymbiosis.
   C. mistletoe.
   D. exosymbiosis.
   E. phoresy.

9. Bennett first used the word "symbiosis" to describe the mutualistic relationship of:

   A. lichens.
   B. coral reefs.
   C. unlike organisms.
   D. lactobacilli

10. A parasite is said to be biotrophic when:

    A. it survives on a dead host.
    B. it relies on the host's survival.
    C. it lives within the host's body.
    D. it feeds on the host's blood.

11. The biologist Lynn Margulis contradicts Darwin's notion of evolution because the latter assumes co-operation, interaction, and mutual dependence among organisms.

    A. Both the statement and reason are correct and related.
    B. Both the statement and the reason are correct but NOT related.
    C. The statement is correct, but the reason is NOT.
    D. The statement is NOT correct, but the reason is correct.
    E. NEITHER the statement NOR the reason is correct.

12. Adaptive speciation caused the flowering plants and their pollinators to undergo the following developments EXCEPT one. Which one is the EXCEPTION?

   A. Specialized morphology of pollinators
   B. Diversity of the plant species
   C. Pollination by insects, bats, or birds
   D. Obligate relationship of some plants and insects

13. Eukaryotes include the following EXCEPT:

   A. plants.
   B. animals.
   C. fungi.
   D. bacteria.
   E. protists.

14. An obligate symbiotic relationship is described to be that:

   A. both symbionts cannot live on their own.
   B. both symbionts can but do not have to live with the other organism.
   C. one of the two symbionts can live on its own.
   D. one of the symbionts lives on the other.
   E. both symbionts are protective of the other.

15. The definition of symbiosis is controversial among scientists because some believe that symbiosis should refer to all types of persistent biological interactions.

   A. Both the statement and reason are correct and related.
   B. Both the statement and the reason are correct but NOT related.
   C. The statement is correct, but the reason is NOT.
   D. The statement is NOT correct, but the reason is correct.
   E. NEITHER the statement NOR the reason is correct.

16. Who is the first scientist to provide a definition for symbiosis?

   A. Lynn Margulis
   B. Bennett
   C. Charles Darwin
   D. Heinrich Anton de Bary
   E. Dorion Sagan

17. Parasitic symbioses involve only relationships in which one member of the association lives within the host's body.

Half of all animals have at least one parasitic phase in their life cycles.

A. Both statements are true.
B. Both statements are false.
C. The first sentence is true while the second sentence is false.
D. The first sentence is false while the second sentence is true.

18. Any symbiotic relationship in which one symbiont lives within the tissues of the other, either in the intracellular or extracellular space is known as:

A. phoresy.
B. inquilinism.
C. metabiosis.
D. endosymbiosis.
E. endoparasitism

If time remains, you may review your work. If your allotted time (20 minutes) is complete, please proceed to the Answer Key.

RC Mini Test 2 Answer Key

1. C	7. A	13. D
2. A	8. D	14. A
3. C	9. A	15. A
4. C	10. B	16. D
5. D	11. C	17. D
6. E	12. C	18. D

RC Mini Test 2 Explanations and Strategies

1.   Question Type: *Application Question*
     Strategies: *SI, OA; P9*

The first sentence in Paragraph 9 defines "amensalism" as the type of symbiotic relationship where one species is inhibited or completely destroyed while the other one is unaffected. The example given in this question closely matches the situation of the sapling and the mature tree, cited in Paragraph 9. Although the herons' existence eventually caused damage to the understory vegetation, the herons in return neither benefited nor got harmed from the lost vegetation. Therefore, the correct answer is C.

(A) Commensalism is roughly the opposite of this, i.e., one species benefits and the other is not significantly harmed or helped. This is also unlike (B) parasitism, where one member in the relationship benefits from either the existence or annihilation of another. On the other hand, (D) ectosymbiosis refers to a symbiotic relationship in which the symbiont feeds on the body surface of the host. This cannot be the correct answer because the herons do not live or feed on the vegetation.

2.   Question Type: *Evaluation Question*
     Strategy: *SaL; P5 last 2 sentences*

Cue words in the statements such as the shrimp being "vulnerable to predators" and the goby fish touches the shrimp with its tail "to warn" strongly suggest that their relationship is based on protection. The context of the paragraph likewise alludes to symbiotic relationships that work around protection.

3. Question Type: *Evaluation Question*
   Strategies: *OA, prior knowledge; P3 S2 and last sentence*

   Contextual clues in Paragraph 3 suggest that rhizobia, Frankia, bacterial endosymbionts provide nutrients (benefits) to their hosts while lactobacilli are generally known as "good" (in the biological context, "mutually beneficial") bacteria. Lice, on the other hand, are parasites and considered as pests – therefore, NOT "good."

4. Question Type: *Evaluation Question (Implication)*
   Strategies: *SaL or OA, PoE, attention to details; P1 S1*

   What makes this question tricky is that the passage offers several definitions of the term "symbiosis." However, A is a definition merely given by Heinrich Anton de Bary as indicated in P1 S3; D is only one of the opinions about symbiosis by some scientists, according to P1 last sentence; and E is loosely a definition from Bennett in P1 S2. This narrows down the choice between B and C. One easy way to determine the best option is to quickly and smartly locate the most conclusive statement that describes "symbiosis." This can be found in P4 S2, "Generally, only lifelong interactions involving close physical and biochemical contact can properly be considered symbiotic." This closely points to C. B, on the other hand, offers a very general definition.

   Another strategy would be to infer how symbiosis mainly works in the various rela-

tionships described in the different paragraphs and then choose the most inclusive definition among the answer choices: C.

5. Question Type: *Application*
   Strategies: *OA/paraphrasing; P6*

   The example in this question is similar to the case of the siboglinid tube worms and symbiotic bacteria discussed in Paragraph 6. The relationship illustrated refers to obligate mutualism: both symbionts entirely depend on each other for survival (P2 S1).

   The other answers are wrong based on each of their definitions:
   (A) Inquilinism pertains to a relationship between two living organisms where one benefits through housing without causing harm or profiting the other either.
   (B) Necrotrophic parasitism is a kind of parasitism that eventually kills the host.
   (C) Biotrophic parasitism only benefits the parasite for as long as the host is alive.
   (E) Facultative mutualism means that both members of the relationship can but do not have to live with the other.

6. Question Type: *Application Question*
   Strategy: *SI or OA; P2, P7, P8*

   Inquilinism is a form of commensalism described as a relationship between two living organisms where one benefits through physical shelter (housing) while the other is not significantly harmed or helped. This type of symbiotic interaction fits the description of an orchid to its host. (A) Ectoparasitism is a close choice. However, ectoparasites live on the surface of their host primarily for nourishment and in the process, cause harm. The other options are off-tangent.

7. Question Type: *True False Statement (Two Statements)*
    Strategies: *SaL, attention to details; P10*

    The first statement is almost verbatim of the first half of P10 S1: "While historically, symbiosis has received less attention than other interactions such as predation or competition. . ." The second statement is a paraphrase of the second half of P10 S2 and S3.

8. Question Type: *Recall*
    Strategy: *SaL; P3 S3*

9. Question Type: *Recall*
    Strategy: *SaL; P1 S2*

10. Question Type: *Recall*
    Strategy: *SaL; P8 S3*

11. Question Type: *True False Statements (Statement and Reason)*
    Strategies: *SI, attention to details; P11 S2*

    The information provided in the reason is reversed.

12. Question Type: *Exception/Negative Question*
    Strategies: *SI, PoE, never lose sight of the question; P12*

    Options A, B, and D are simple paraphrase of the information found in P12 S4 and S5. Pollination by insects, bats, or birds, on the other hand, is not an offshoot of adaptive speciation but rather, a "standard" activity or function of pollinators. The question is specifically asking for the developments, which arose from adaptive speciation, in the flowering plants and their pollinators – not what each already does. Therefore, the answer is C.

13. Question Type: *Exception/Negative Question*
    Strategies: *SaL, PoE; P10 S2*

    In P10 S2, the eukaryotes are specifically identified in a parenthesis to include plants, animals, fungi, and protists. Nowhere in the passage indicates bacteria as a eukaryote.

14. Question Type: *Recall*
    Strategy: *SaL; P2 S1*

15. Question Type: *True False Statement (Statement and Reason)*
    Strategy: *SaL; P1 last 2 sentences*

16. Question Type: *Recall*
    Strategies: *SaL, PoE; P1 S3*

    Bennett was the first to use the term "symbiosis," not define it. Dorion Sagan and Lynn Margulis are the ones who said that "life did not take over the globe by combat, but by networking." Charles Darwin was only mentioned in the passage in relation to Margulis' contention about the theory of evolution.

17. Question Type: *True False Statements (Two Statements)*
    Strategies: *SaL, PoE, attention to details; P8 S2 and S5*

The first statement presents an incomplete definition of parasitic symbioses, which should include endoparasitism (living within a host's body), ectoparasitism (living on the surface of a host), necrotrophic parasitism (killing the host) and biotrophic parasitism (relying on the host's survival).

18. Question Type: *Recall*
    Strategy: *SaL, P3 S1*

Would you like to discuss any of the answers
or strategies in this section?
Go to www.dat-prep.com/forum to share and learn.

RC Mini Test 3

The following is a sample mini test which is comparable to the level of difficulty required for the Reading Comprehension Test of the DAT. Please note that this sample would roughly be 1/3 of the actual Reading Comprehension Test portion of the DAT.

You have 20 minutes to complete this portion of the DAT Mini Test; the actual test is 60 minutes. Please time yourself accordingly.

> BEGIN ONLY WHEN YOUR TIMER IS READY.

Passage 3

Empirical Science

(1). A scientist, whether theorist or experimenter, puts forward statements, or systems of statements, and tests them step by step. In the field of the empirical sciences, more particularly, he constructs hypotheses, or systems of theories, and tests them against experience by observation and experiment. I suggest that it is the task of the logic of scientific discovery, or the logic of knowledge, to give a logical analysis of this procedure; that is, to analyze the method of the empirical sciences.

(2). But what are these "methods of the empirical sciences"? And what do we call "empirical science"?

(3). According to a widely accepted view — to be opposed in this book — the empirical sciences can be characterized by the fact that they use "inductive methods," as they are called. According to this view, the logic of scientific discovery would be identical with inductive logic, i.e. with the logical analysis of these inductive methods.

(4). It is usual to call an inference "inductive" if it passes from singular statements (sometimes also called "particular" statements), such as accounts of the results of observations or experiments, to universal statements, such as hypotheses or theories.

(5). Now it is far from obvious, from a logical point of view, that we are justified in inferring universal statements from singular ones, no matter how numerous; for any conclusion drawn in this way may always turn out to be false: no matter how many instances of white swans we may have observed, this does not justify the conclusion that all swans are white.

(6). The question whether inductive inferences are justified, or under what conditions, is known as the problem of induction. The problem of induction may also be formulated as the question of the validity or the truth of universal statements which are based on experience, such as the hypotheses and theoretical systems of the empirical sciences. For many people believe that the truth of these universal statements is "known by experience"; yet it is clear that an account of an experience — of an observation or the result of an experiment — can in the first place be only a singular statement and not a universal one. Accordingly, people who say of a universal statement that we know its truth from experience usually mean that the truth of this universal statement can somehow be reduced to the truth of singular ones, and that these singular ones are known by experience to be true; which amounts to saying that the universal statement is based on inductive inference. Thus to ask whether there are natural laws known to be true appears to be only another way of asking whether inductive inferences are logically justified.

(7). Yet if we want to find a way of justifying inductive inferences, we must first of all try to establish a principle of induction. A principle of induction would be a statement with the help of which we could put inductive inferences into a logically acceptable form. In the eyes of the upholders of inductive logic, a principle of induction is of supreme importance for scientific method: ". . . this principle," says Reichenbach, "determines the truth of scientific theories. To eliminate it from science would mean nothing less than to deprive science of the power to decide the truth or falsity of its theories. Without it, clearly, science would no longer have the right to distinguish its theories from the fanciful and arbitrary creations of the poet's mind."

(8). Now this principle of induction cannot be a purely logical truth like a tautology or an analytic statement. Indeed, if there were such a thing as a purely logical principle of induction, there would be no problem of induction; for in this case, all inductive inferences would have to be regarded as purely logical or tautological transformations, just like inferences in deductive logic. Thus the principle of induction must be a synthetic statement; that is, a statement whose negation is not self-contradictory but logically possible. So the question arises why such a principle should be accepted at all, and how we can justify its acceptance on rational grounds.

(9). Some who believe in inductive logic are anxious to point out, with Reichenbach, that "the principle of induction is unreservedly accepted by the whole of science and that no man can seriously doubt this principle in everyday life either." Yet even supposing this were the case — for after all, "the whole of science" might err — I should still contend that a principle of induction is superfluous, and that it must lead to logical inconsistencies.

(10). That inconsistencies may easily arise in connection with the principle of induction should have been clear from the work of Hume, also, that they can be avoided, if at all, only with difficulty. For the principle of induction must be a universal statement in its turn. Thus if we try to regard its truth as known from experience, then the very same problems which occasioned its introduction will arise all over again. To justify it, we should have to employ inductive inferences; and to justify these we should have to assume an inductive principle of a higher order; and so on. Thus the attempt to base the principle of induction on experience breaks down, since it must lead to an infinite regress.

(11). Kant tried to force his way out of this difficulty by taking the principle of induction (which he formulated as the "principle of universal causation") to be "a priori valid." But I do not think that his ingenious attempt to provide an a priori justification for synthetic statements was successful.

(12). My own view is that the various difficulties of inductive logic here sketched are insurmountable. So also, I fear, are those inherent in the doctrine, so widely current today, that inductive inference, although not "strictly valid," can attain some degree of "reliability" or of "probability." According to this doctrine, inductive inferences are "probable inferences." "We have described," says Reichenbach, "the principle of induction as the means whereby science decides upon truth. To be more exact, we should say that it serves to decide upon probability. For it is not given to science to reach either truth or falsity . . . but scientific statements can only attain continuous degrees of probability whose unattainable upper and lower limits are truth and falsity." At this stage I can disregard the fact that the believers in inductive logic entertain an idea of probability that I shall later reject as highly unsuitable for their own purposes. I can do so because the difficulties mentioned are not even touched by an appeal to probability. For if a certain degree of probability is to be assigned to statements based on inductive inference, then this will have to be justified by invoking a new principle of induction, appropriately modified. And this new principle in its turn will have to be justified, and so on. Nothing is gained, moreover, if the principle of induction, in its turn, is taken not as "true" but only as "probable." In short, like every other form of inductive logic, the logic of probable inference, or "probability logic," leads either to an infinite regress, or to the doctrine of apriorism.

(13). The theory to be developed in the following pages stands directly opposed to all attempts to operate with the ideas of inductive logic. It might be described as the theory of the deductive method of testing, or as the view that a hypothesis can only be empirically tested — and only after it has been advanced.

(14). Before I can elaborate this view (which might be called "deductivism," in contrast to "inductivism") I must first make clear the distinction between the psychology of knowledge which deals with empirical facts, and the logic of knowledge which is concerned only with logical relations. For the belief in inductive logic is largely due to a confusion of psychological problems with epistemological ones. It may be worth noticing, by the way, that this confusion spells trouble not only for the logic of knowledge but for its psychology as well.

- from Karl Popper's *Logic of Scientific Discovery*

1. The problem of induction is best represented by which of the following equations?

A. X = Z always
B. X = Z many times, so X must be the same as Z
C. X never equals Z, so X is unique and apart from Z
D. X is sometimes Z, but only in certain situations
E. X is derived from Z on the basis of logic

2. Of the following, which is tested by a scientist against experience with observation and experiment?

A. Inductive logic
B. Deductive logic
C. Empirical sciences
D. Hypotheses and theories
E. None of the above

3. The idea of an "infinite regress" results from the idea that a theory is:

A. after experience.
B. before experience.
C. deductively sound.
D. inductively inferred.
E. a priori.

4. With which of the following statements would the author of the passage agree?

A. Deductive logic should be preferred over inductive logic.
B. The methods of empirical science are marked by circular reasoning.
C. Inductive logic is questionable and suspect.
D. Tautological statements support observation and hypotheses.
E. Scientists need to justify inductive inferences.

5. Based on usage in this passage, which of the following best defines "empirical"?

A. Arbitrary
B. Inferable
C. Falsifiable
D. Observable
E. More than one of the above

6. Which of the following analogies best represents the idea of infinite regress?

A. A bridge connected to another bridge
B. A circle within another circle
C. A snake eating its own tail (uberous)
D. A mirror turned towards another mirror
E. A vessel with many interconnected chambers

7. Inductive logic, by its nature, supposedly passes from the "singular event" to:

A. the hypothetical derived.
B. the a priori established.
C. the universally true.
D. the testable observation.
E. the experimental deduced.

8. The author's tone and type of audience are which of the following terms?

A. Critical - Scientific Community
B. Arcane - General Populace
C. Careful - Students
D. Witty - Academic
E. Profound - Logicians

9. The principle of induction serves to decide upon probability in science because it is given to science to reach either truth or falsity.

A. Both the statement and reason are correct and related.
B. Both the statement and the reason are correct but NOT related.
C. The statement is correct but the reason is NOT.
D. The statement is NOT correct, but the reason is correct.
E. NEITHER the statement NOR the reason is correct.

10. Reichenbach organizes a principle of induction around:

    A. the establishment of logical inferences.
    B. social consensus of the scientific community.
    C. logically derived a priori formulations.
    D. other inductive tautologies.
    E. None of the above

11. Of the following, which according to the passage are the functions of the principle of induction?

    1. Characterizes empirical science as tautological
    2. Justifies inductive inferences as a logical form
    3. Determines the truth of scientific theories
    4. Distinguishes science from creative art

    A. All of the above
    B. 2, 3 and 4 only
    C. 2 and 3 only
    D. 3 only
    E. 4 only

12. The problem of induction is basically:

    A. how to refine this logical process.
    B. how to avoid this process in favor of deduction.
    C. whether its applications are logically faulty.
    D. whether inductive inferences are justified or under what conditions.
    E. how there is an inherent contradiction in inductive inferences.

13. In the last paragraph, the statement to "make clear the distinction between the psychology of knowledge which deals with empirical facts, and the logic of knowledge which is concerned only with logical relations" can be inferred to be the author's juxtaposition between:

    A. what is observable and what is testable.
    B. what is hypothetical and what is logically sound.
    C. what is testable and what is inductive.
    D. what is observable and what is logically sound.
    E. what is inductive and what is universally true.

14. What is the task of the logic of scientific discovery?

A. To analyze the method of empirical sciences

B. To put forward statements and test them step by step

C. To test scientific theories against experience by observation and experiment

D. To employ inductive logic

E. All of the above

15. Which of the following is the best description of a synthetic statement?

A. A statement based on experience

B. A universal statement based on inductive inference

C. The power to decide the truth or falsity of a theory

D. A statement whose negation is not self-contradictory but logically possible

E. A purely logical or tautological transformation

If time remains, you may review your work. If your allotted time (20 minutes) is complete, please proceed to the Answer Key.

RC Mini Test 3 Answer Key

1. B	6. D	11. B
2. D	7. C	12. D
3. D	8. A	13. D
4. C	9. C	14. A
5. D	10. B	15. D

RC Mini Test 3 Explanations and Strategies

1. Question Type: *Evaluation Question (Main Idea)*
   Strategy: *OA*

   The whole passage is about how inductive logic compiles on examples in order to move from the singular examples to the universal. A is incorrect because that would posit the problem of induction as an exact correspondence between entities or phenomena. C is also incorrect because this equation suggests an inequality, subtraction or difference of phenomena or entities. This is closer to deduction, not induction. D is incorrect because it gives X a contextually determined essence. E is a made up phrase, simply made to distract the test taker.

2. Question Type: *Recall*
   Strategy: *SaL; P1 S2*

3. Question Type: *Evaluation Question (Implication)*
   Strategy: *SaL or OA, P10 last 2 sentences, P12 last sentence*

   The idea of infinite regress can be inferred based on the author's discussion in Paragraph 10: a theory supported through induction must be inductively inferred as well, resulting to an endless chain of induction. After Experience or A Posteriori, as well as Before Experience or A Priori, are related but not as specific to the idea of infinite regress. C is quite the contrary, and can be ruled out.

4. Question Type: *Evaluation Question (Tone and Main Idea)*
   Strategies: *OA, attention to details in P3*

Early in the passage, the author expresses his opposition to the inductive method: "According to a widely accepted view — to be opposed in this book — the empirical sciences can be characterized by the fact that they use 'inductive methods'." This statement would readily give a clear hint of the author's tone – that of contradiction, which is closest to viewing inductive logic as "questionable and suspect."

Another strategy is to paraphrase the main idea of each significant paragraph in order to have a clear outline of the author's overall point.

(1). I suggest that it is the task of the logic of scientific discovery, or the logic of knowledge, to give a logical analysis of this procedure; that is, to analyze the method of the empirical sciences.

(3). The author explicitly contradicts the inductive method.

(4). Induction starts with the specific "particular" or "singular" to the general or "universal."

(5). This method is not justified because "any conclusion drawn in this way may always turn out to be false."

(6). The problem of the inductive method is that the truth of the universal statements is questionable and cannot be justified because they are based on a particular observation or a singular result of an experiment. In other words, a universal statement cannot be justified by a singular experience or event.

(7). In order to justify the inductive method, a principle of induction must first be established. (A principle of induction would be a statement with the help of which we could put inductive inferences into a logically acceptable form.)

(8). Ideally, a principle of induction must present a synthetic statement - a statement whose negation is not self-contradictory but logically possible.

(9). The author believes that a principle of induction is superfluous (unnecessary), and that it must lead to logical inconsistencies. On the other hand, Reichenbach asserts that "the principle of induction is unreservedly accepted by the whole of science and that no man can seriously doubt this principle in everyday life either."

(10). The principle of induction is prone to infinite regress.

(11). Kant fails to provide an a priori justification for synthetic statements.

(12). Inductive logic is problematic in several ways: inductive inference, although not "strictly valid," can attain some degree of "reliability" or of "probability"; "probability logic," leads either to an infinite regress, or to the doctrine of apriorism.

(13). The author introduces the idea of deductivism.

(14). The author distinguishes his idea of "the psychology of knowledge which deals with empirical facts (from) the logic of knowledge which is concerned only with logical relations.

The preceding brief notes clearly indicate that the author's concern in this excerpt is questioning the validity of inductive logic. Therefore, the most reasonable answer to this question would be C.

The author does mention his preference to deductivism over inductivism. However, this is not elaborated in the passage. A, then, would not be an accurate answer. (B) Circular reasoning in empirical science is not asserted in the passage either.

Although tautology in relation to logic is mentioned, the idea that (D) tautological statements support observation and hypotheses is off-tangent in the context of the passage. Lastly, the author does not seek that (E) "scientists need to justify inductive inferences." Rather, he dismisses the use of such method as resulting to infinite regress.

5. Question Type: *Evaluation Question (Implication)*
   Strategies: *OA, PoE; P1, P3, P4, P6*

(A) Arbitrary is the term used by the author to describe poetic creations. This can be readily eliminated then. On the other hand, inferring from paragraphs that refer to "empirical" or "empirical science" often suggests the following key ideas: "experience by observation and experiment" (P1 S2); "the empirical sciences can be characterized by the fact that they use 'inductive methods'" (P3 S1), correlating to the notion in Paragraph 4 that induction entails "observations or experiments." These lead to D (observable) as the best choice.

Although (B) inference is repeatedly mentioned in the passage, this is used in reference to the inductive method per se, not empirical science. (C) Falsifiable is an element of theory, which limits scope, i.e., the theory does not include everything, thus this is prescriptive evaluation and reservations of a given theory, not a definition in itself. E can thus be eliminated as well.

6. Question Type: *Application Question*
   Strategies: *OA/paraphrasing, PoE; P10 and P12*

Since "infinite regress" is the idea that inductive logic which is inferred is based on an inference, and that inference is based on another inference and so on, the best analogy would be (D) of a mirror turned towards a mirror reproducing its own representation. The notion of (C) a snake eating its own tail, comes close to representing the tautological reasoning sometimes used to support inductive modes of logic: Premise = CLAIM = Premise. However, the idea of something eating up its own self suggests an end, therefore not "infinite."

The analogy of (A) a bridge connected to another bridge is also close but is only limited to one extension – not one after another. (B)

A circle within a circle suggests related but separate inferences – not a continuation. This is the same with the idea in E. These make all the other options incorrect.

7. Question Type: *Evaluation Question (Implication); Recall*
   Strategies: *Paraphrasing, SaL; P4*

   This question is merely a paraphrase of the general idea found in Paragraph 4, which states induction starts with the specific – "particular" or "singular" – to the general or "universal."

8. Question Type: *Evaluation Question (Tone)*
   Strategy: *SI*

   The author makes clear from the beginning that he is opposed to the idea of inductive logic. He then devotes a majority of his succeeding discussions in pointing out the problems of induction. He is therefore, critical. In addition, constant references to empirical science and experiments make this passage generally suited for the scientific community, which can include students or the academic audience and logicians as well.

   However, (D) witty does not characterize the tone of the author. (C) Careful and (E) profound may be reasonable descriptions of the quality of the author's writing, but they are not as encompassing and specific.

   (B) Arcane connotes ambiguous or difficult to understand, which is illogical to have something written in this language to be meant

for the general populace. Thus B is wrong.

9. Question Type: *True False Statements (Statement and Reason)*
   Strategy: *SaL; P12 S4 to S6*

10. Question Type: *Recall*
    Strategies: *SaL, attention to details; P9 S1*

    As the passage states in a quote from Reichenbach, "the principle of induction is unreservedly accepted by the whole of science and that no man can seriously doubt this principle in everyday life." This amounts to a social consensus of the inductive method. Answer A is nonsense. E (None of the Above) can be ruled out. D may be true, in the idea of infinite regress, but the question states "the principle of induction." C is more or less philoso-babble constructed in the answers to distract the test taker.

11. Question Type: *Recall; Evaluation (Implication)*
    Strategies: *SI, paraphrasing; P7 and P8 S1*

    This question pertains to the discussion of establishing a principle of induction found in Paragraph 7. According to the author, "a principle of induction would be a statement with the help of which we could put inductive inferences into a logically acceptable form" (Statement 2). For Reichenbach, this principle "determines the truth of scientific theories" (Statement 3) and "distinguish(es) (scientific) theories from the fanciful and arbitrary creations of the poet's mind" (Statement 4).

P8 S1 would eliminate Statement 1: "Now this principle of induction cannot be a purely logical truth like a tautology or an analytic statement." Therefore, the best answer is B.

12. Question Type: *Recall*
Strategy: *SaL; P6 S1*

13. Question Type: *Evaluation (Implication)*
Strategies: *OA/paraphrasing, inference*

This question requires clearly understanding what "empirical" mainly connotes in the passage. As already determined and explained in Question No. 5, empirical or empirical facts would indicate something "observable." Additionally, the author makes a significant remark in Paragraph 8 that for a method, such as that of induction, to work, a synthetic statement must result: one that is logically valid or possible. Hence, the correct answer is D: the author juxtaposes "what is observable (empirical facts) and what is logically sound (logical relations)."

A is incorrect because logical relations is not indicated in the passage as "testable." B is also

wrong because hypothetical does not directly characterize an "empirical fact." Hypothesis is only part of this process. C is primarily incorrect because of the term "induction" being correlated to logic. The author explicitly opposes this view. E sounds correct; however, it must be noted that the author has not established the concept of logic to be "universally true." Therefore, E is an erroneous statement.

14. Question Type: *Recall*
Strategy: *SaL; P1 last sentence*

The two key phrases here are "empirical facts" and "logical relations" - meaning "observations" and "logic as a system of itself." Therefore, an analysis of the method of empirical sciences – as explicitly stated in the last sentence of Paragraph 1 – is the best answer. B and C are corollaries or peripheral statements that simply relate to the passage in general while D goes against the main idea of the author.

15. Question Type: *Recall*
Strategy: *SaL; P8 S3*

Would you like to discuss any of the answers
or strategies in this section?
Go to www.dat-prep.com/forum to share and learn.

RC Mini Test 4

The following is a sample mini test which is comparable to the level of difficulty required for the Reading Comprehension Test of the DAT. Please note that this sample would roughly be 1/3 of the actual Reading Comprehension Test portion of the DAT.

You have 20 minutes to complete this portion of the DAT Mini Test; the actual test is 60 minutes. Please time yourself accordingly.

> BEGIN ONLY WHEN YOUR TIMER IS READY.

Passage 4

Macroscopic Parameters

(1). Macroscopic processes appear to be temporally "directed" in some sense. Systems spontaneously evolve to future equilibrium states, but they do not spontaneously evolve away from equilibrium states. The nature of this directedness raises many questions in the foundations of philosophy and science.

(2). Thermodynamics is the science that describes much of the time-asymmetric behavior found in the world. This entry's first task, consequently, is to show how thermodynamics treats temporally 'directed' behavior. It then concentrates on the following two questions: (1) What is the origin of the thermodynamic asymmetry in time? In a world possibly governed by time-symmetric laws, how should we understand the time-asymmetric laws of thermodynamics? (2) Does the thermodynamic time asymmetry explain the other temporal asymmetries? Does it account, for instance, for the fact that we know more about the past than the future? The discussion thus divides between thermodynamics being an explanandum or explanans. In the former case the answer will be found in philosophy of physics; in the latter case it will be found in metaphysics, epistemology, and other fields, though in each case there will be blurring between the disciplines.

(3). Consider the following.

Place some chlorine gas in a small closed flask into the corner of a room. Set it up so that an automaton will remove its cover in 1 minute. Now we know what to do: run. Chlorine is poison, and furthermore, we know the gas will spread reasonably quickly through its available volume. The chlorine originally in equilibrium in the flask will, upon being freed, 'relax' to a new equilibrium.

(4). Or less dramatically:

Place an iron bar over a flame for half an hour. Place another one in a freezer for the same duration. Remove them and place them against one another. Within a short time the hot one will 'lose its heat' to the cold one. The new combined two-bar system will settle to a new equilibrium, one intermediate between the cold and hot bar's original temperatures. Eventually the bars will together settle to roughly room temperature.

(5). These are two examples of a tendency of systems to spontaneously evolve to equilibrium; but there are indefinitely more examples in all manner of substance. The physics first used to systematically describe such processes is thermodynamics.

(6). First developed in S. Carnot's Reflections on the Motive Power of Fire 1824, the science of classical thermodynamics is intimately associated with the industrial revolution. Most of the results responsible for the science originated from the practice of engineers trying to improve steam engines. Begun in France and England in the late eighteenth and early nineteenth centuries, the science quickly spread throughout Europe. By the mid-nineteenth century, Clausius in Germany and Thomson (later Lord Kelvin) in England had developed the theory in great detail.

(7). Thermodynamics is a 'phenomenal' science, in the sense that the variables of the science range over macroscopic parameters such as temperature and volume. Whether the microphysics underlying these variables are motive atoms in the void or an imponderable fluid is largely irrelevant to this science. The developers of the theory both prided themselves on this fact and at the same time worried about it. Clausius, for instance, was one of the first to speculate that heat consisted solely of the motion of particles (without an ether), for it made the equivalence of heat with mechanical work less surprising. However, as was common, he kept his "ontological" beliefs separate from his statement of the principles of thermodynamics because he didn't wish to (in his words) "taint" the latter with the speculative character of the former.

(8). A treatment of thermodynamics naturally begins with the statements it takes to be laws of nature. These laws are founded upon observations of relationships between particular macroscopic parameters and they are justified by the fact they are empirically adequate. No further justification of these laws is to be found — at this stage — from the details of microphysics. Rather, stable, counterfactual-supporting generalizations about macroscopic features are enshrined as law. The typical textbook treatment of thermodynamics describes some basic concepts, states the laws in a more or less rough way and then proceeds to derive the concepts of temperature and entropy and the various thermodynamic equations of state. It is worth remarking, however, that in the last fifty years the subject has been presented with a degree of mathematical rigor not previously achieved. Originating from the early axiomatization by Carathéodory in 1909, the development of 'rational thermodynamics' has clarified the concepts and logic of classical thermodynamics to a degree not generally appreciated. There now exist many quite different, mathematically exact approaches to thermodynamics, each starting with different primitive kinds and/or observational regularities as axioms. (For a popular presentation of a recent axiomatization, *see* Lieb and Yngvason 2000.)

(9). In the traditional approach classical thermodynamics has two laws, the second of which is our main focus. (Readers may have heard of a 'third law' as well, but it was added later and is not relevant to the present discussion.) The first law expresses the conservation of energy. The law uses the concept of the internal energy of a system, U, which is a function of variables such as volume. For thermally isolated (adiabatic) systems—think of systems such as coffee in a thermos—the law states that this function, U, is such that the work W delivered to a system's surroundings is compensated by a loss of internal energy, i.e., $dW = -dU$. When Joule and others showed that mechanical work and heat were interconvertible, consistency with the principle of energy conservation demanded that heat, Q, considered as a different form of energy, be taken into account. For non-isolated systems we extend the law as $dQ = dU + dW$, where dQ is the differential of the amount of heat added to the system (in a reversible manner).

(10). The conservation of energy tells us nothing about temporally asymmetric behavior. In particular, it doesn't follow from the first law that interacting systems quickly tend to approach equilibrium (a state where the values of the macroscopic variables remain approximately stable), and once achieved, never leave this state. It is perfectly consistent with the first law that systems in equilibrium leave equilibrium. Since this tendency of systems cannot be derived from the First Law, another law is needed. Although Carnot was the first to state it, the formulations of Kelvin and Clausius are standard:

(11). Kelvin's Second Law: There is no thermodynamic process whose sole effect is to transform heat extracted from a source at uniform temperature completely into work.

(12). Clausius' Second Law: There is no thermodynamic process whose sole effect is to extract a quantity of heat from a colder reservoir and deliver it to a hotter reservoir.

(13). Kelvin's version is essentially the same as the version arrived at by both Carnot and Planck, whereas Clausius' version differs from these in a few ways.

(14). Clausius' version transparently rules out anti-thermodynamic behavior such as a hot iron bar extracting heat from a neighboring cold iron bar. The cool bar cannot give up a quantity of heat to the warmer bar (without something else happening). Kelvin's statement is perhaps less obvious. It originates in an observation about steam engines, namely, that heat energy is a 'poor' grade of energy. Consider a gas-filled cylinder with a frictionless piston holding the gas down at one end. If we put a flame under the cylinder, the gas will expand and the piston can perform work, e.g., it might move a ball. However, we can never convert the heat energy straight into work without some other effect occurring. In this case, the gas occupies a larger volume.

(15). In 1854 Clausius introduced the notion of the 'equivalence value' of a transformation, a concept that is the ancestor of the modern day concept of entropy. Later in 1865 Clausius coined the term 'entropy' for a similar concept (the word derives from the Greek word for transformation). The entropy of a state A, $S(A)$ is defined as the integral $S(A) = \int_O^A dQ/T$ over a reversible transformation, where O is some arbitrary fixed state. For A to have an entropy, the transformation from O to A must be quasistatic, i.e., a succession of equilibrium states. Continuity considerations then imply that the initial and final states O and A must also be equilibrium states. In terms of entropy, the Second Law states that in a transformation from equilibrium state A to equilibrium state B, the inequality $S(B) - S(A)$ is greater than or equal to the $\int_B^A dQ/T$. Loosely put, for realistic systems, this implies that in the spontaneous evolution of a thermally closed system the entropy can never decrease and that it attains its maximum value for states at equilibrium. We are invited to think of the Second Law as driving the gas to its new, higher entropy equilibrium state. Using this concept of entropy, thermodynamics is able to capture an extraordinary range of phenomena under one simple law. Remarkably, whether they are gases filling their available volumes, two iron bars in contact coming to the same temperature, or milk mixing in your coffee, they all have an observable property in common: their entropy increases. Coupled with the First Law, the Second Law is remarkably powerful. It appears that all classical thermodynamical behavior can be derived from these two simple statements (Penrose 1970).

1. Macroscopic parameters refer to the philosophy underlying thermodynamics. Microscopic physics refers to empirical variables, such as temperature and volume.

    A. The first statement is true. The second statement is false.
    B. The first statement is false. The second statement is true
    C. Both statements are true.
    D. Both statements are false.

2. The notion of thermodynamics originated from:

    A. general studies by early physicists.

    B. efforts by engineers to improve the steam engine.

    C. chemists noticing certain paradoxes in experimentation

    D. studies in ways to make coal industries more efficient.

    E. philosophers speculating on the nature of time.

3. What is meant by the phrase in the first paragraph: "Systems spontaneously evolve to future equilibrium states, but they do not spontaneously evolve away from equilibrium states." What is the BEST inference to be made from the list below?

    A. That systems are paradoxical.

    B. Equilibrium is marked by a duality.

    C. The evolution of systems to and away from equilibrium is spatially oriented.

    D. Spontaneous evolution of systems is marked by equilibrium.

    E. System evolutions to and away from equilibrium is marked by two modes of time.

4. The BEST alternative title of this passage would be:

    A. Systems Evolution and Thermodynamics.

    B. A History of the Second Law of Thermodynamics.

    C. Equilibrium and Systems Theory.

    D. Thermodynamic Asymmetry of Time.

    E. The Properties of the Second Law of Thermodynamics.

5. An *explanandum* to the questions raised by the author can be found in the philosophy of physics.

   An *explanans* to the questions raised by the author can be found in the science of physics.

    A. The first statement is true. The second statement is false.

    B. The first statement is false. The second statement is true

    C. Both statements are true.

    D. Both the statements are false.

6. The author's main thesis is to describe:

   A. thermodynamics and philosophy.
   B. the nature of the Second Law of Thermodynamics.
   C. thermodynamics and asymmetric temporality.
   D. thermodynamics and equilibrium.
   E. macroscopic and microscopic processes in thermodynamics.

7. Which of the following was NOT involved in developing the laws of thermodynamics in the eighteenth and nineteenth centuries? Which person is the EXCEPTION?

   A. Carnot
   B. Carathéodory
   C. Lord Kelvin
   D. Clausius
   E. Thomson

8. To which of the following does the first law of thermodynamics generally refer to?

   A. Principles of Equilibrium
   B. The parameters of temperature and volume
   C. The conservation of energy
   D. Constants of heat and time
   E. Evolution of systems

9. Clausius' notion of "equivalence value of a transformation" is a modern day concept of:

   A. temperature-volume ratios.
   B. the conservation of energy.
   C. equilibrium.
   D. constants of heat.
   E. entropy.

10. What can be inferred to be the BEST definition of thermodynamic "equilibrium"?

   A. The transference valuation between the effects of energy and work
   B. Changed or unchanged properties of a system based on the temporal direction and effect of interactions between energy, pressure, volume, and temperature
   C. A state where volume and temperature values remain stable
   D. A state where an object or system and its surroundings cease to exchange energy in the form of heat
   E. The condition of a system in which macroscopic variables evolve in time

11. Which of the following is the correct definition of Kelvin's Second Law of Thermodynamics? Which is the BEST answer?

   A. There is no thermodynamic process whose sole effect is to extract a quantity of heat from a colder reservoir and deliver it to a hotter reservoir.
   B. There is no thermodynamic process whose sole effect is to transform heat from a colder reservoir and deliver it to a hotter reservoir.
   C. There is no thermodynamic process whose sole effect is to extract a quantity of heat from a source at different temperatures completely into work.
   D. There is no thermodynamic process whose sole effect is to transform heat extracted from a source at uniform temperature completely into work.
   E. There is no thermodynamic process whose sole effect is to transform work extracted from heat constancy solely into energy.

12. The term "entropy" was coined by Clausius in:

   A. 1856.
   B. 1854.
   C. 1909.
   D. 1865.
   E. 1824.

13. Which of the following would not be considered an example of entropy. Which is the EXCEPTION?

   A. Ice melting in a warmer room
   B. Hot coffee eventually getting cooler within an open mug
   C. Water boiling and eventually evaporating into the air
   D. The flow of information in a communication system resulting in a feedback loop
   E. A warm soda poured over cold ice resulting in a fizzing and foaming.

14. Several mathematically exact approaches to thermodynamics now exist because classical thermodynamics has clarified the concepts and logic of rational thermodynamics.

   A. Both the statement and reason are correct and related.
   B. Both the statement and the reason are correct but NOT related.
   C. The statement is correct but the reason is NOT.
   D. The statement is NOT correct, but the reason is correct.
   E. NEITHER the statement NOR the reason is correct.

15. Which of the following in NOT true about the author's discussion of the philosophy of thermodynamics and the physics of thermodynamics? Which is the EXCEPTION?

A. Thermodynamics in a sense prided itself from being "untainted" by speculation.

B. Whether the microphysics underlying these variables are motive atoms in the void or an imponderable fluid is largely irrelevant to this science.

C. A typical textbook treatment of thermodynamics, starts with the simple variables involved, and no further philosophical justification is needed.

D. Clausius himself thought that thermodynamics processes took place within the context of unobservable ether within the system.

E. The early researchers of thermodynamics tended to keep their physical beliefs separate from their ontological beliefs.

16. Which of the following CANNOT be considered a variable in a thermodynamic process?

A. Temperature
B. Volume
C. Protons
D. Energy
E. Pressure

If time remains, you may review your work. If your allotted time (20 minutes) is complete, please proceed to the Answer Key.

RC Mini Test 4 Answer Key

1. D	5. A	9. E	13. D
2. B	6. C	10. C	14. C
3. E	7. B	11. D	15. D
4. D	8. C	12. D	16. C

RC Mini Test 4 Explanations and Strategies

For this Mini Test only, identify the Question Type and/or Strategy that works best for you.

1.   Question Type: _____
     Strategy: *Skimming for Ideas (SI); P7 S1 and S2**

True or false statements appear at least once or twice on every passage in the DAT RC test. This is a concept-oriented question that mostly requires scanning the specified information within the passage or skimming for the general idea. In other cases, it could involve inference skills and some general knowledge in the sciences such as is the case in this question.

Macroscopic parameters refer to variables such as temperature and volume. These do not constitute a philosophy. Therefore, the first statement - "Macroscopic parameters refer to the philosophy underlying thermodynamics." - is false. Similarly, microphysics or microscopic physics, as its name implies, deal with elements

(for example, atoms) that cannot be possibly observed without using a scientific equipment or method. In other words, microphysics cannot refer to empirical variables; therefore, the second statement is also false.

2.   Question Type: _____
     Strategy: *SaL; P6 S2*

This question merely requires recalling and locating information mentioned in a specific paragraph of the passage. This is the most common type of RC question in the DAT. The best strategy here is "scan and locate" (SaL) - very much similar to the "search and destroy" method popularized by a user named "VicViper" in the SDN forums.

The correct answer, **B**, is indicated in the second sentence of Paragraph 6.

3. Question Type: _____
   Strategy: *PoE*

This is an inference type of question that requires you to understand and interpret the concept highlighted in the problem. Some past DAT candidates report having encountered quite a number of this question type while others, only a few to almost none for the entire RC test.

One way to deal with this question is by employing the process of elimination (PoE). Start discarding the most obvious wrong answer, which is **C**. P1 S1 indicates that the evolution of systems is temporally – NOT spatially – "directed." Next is **A**: nothing in the passage suggests or discusses anything about systems being self-contradictory or paradoxical. **B** may sound correct, but the statement in question refers to the evolution of systems rather than the nature of equilibrium. Therefore, **B** is off.

You now have to consider the context surrounding the statement. The prior sentence refers to macroscopic processes within the system to be seemingly directed by time (temporally "directed"). The first two sentences of Paragraph 2 likewise hint at "time" as an important factor in considering system evolutions in thermodynamics. Between **D** and **E**, option **E** has a more encompassing interpretation of the given statement.

4. Question Type: _____
   Strategy: _____

This is another type of inference question, which is typical in the DAT RC.

With questions asking what "the best title" would be for a passage, the easiest approach is to identify the main theme or the author's main purpose. This is quite easy for this passage because the author explicitly states this in the second sentence of Paragraph 2: "This entry's first task, consequently, is to show how thermodynamics treats temporally 'directed' behavior." Likewise, asymmetry of time and time-asymmetric processes are discussed throughout the passage . The best answer is **D**.

5. Question Type: _____
   Strategy: *SaL; P2 last two sentences*

The first statement is almost verbatim of the first half of the last sentence of Paragraph 2. Hence it is true. *Explanans*, on the other hand, is said to be found in the field of metaphysics and epistemology, which are branches of philosophy, NOT science. The second statement is thus false. The correct answer is **A**.

6. Question Type: _____
   Strategy: _____

This question is quite similar to question number 4, and the best hint to the correct answer can be found in P2 S2: "This entry's first task, consequently, is to show how thermodynamics treats temporally 'directed' behavior." The best option is **C**.

7. Question Type: _____
   Strategy: *SaL, SI; P6 S1, P8 S7*

Carnot, Clausius, and Thomson are all mentioned in Paragraph 6 to have contributed in the development of theories in thermodynamics. In the succeeding paragraphs, the author further relates that these personalities went on to develop the laws of thermodynamics. Lord Kelvin (option **C**) is another name that Thomson is known for (P6 last sentence).

On the other hand, Carathéodory originated "axiomatization" in thermodynamics in the early twentieth century – 1909 – not in the eighteenth or nineteenth century. Option **B**, Carathéodory, is the EXCEPTION in the list.

8. Question Type: _____
   Strategy: *SaL; P9 S3*

Sentence 3 of Paragraph 9 explicitly states that "the first law expresses the conservation of energy."

9. Question Type: _____
   Strategy: *SaL; P15 S1*

This question can be easily answered by scanning the passage and locating the information on the first sentence of Paragraph 15: "In 1854 Clausius introduced the notion of the 'equivalence value' of a transformation, a concept that is the ancestor of the modern day concept of entropy."

10. Question Type: _____
    Strategy: *SaL, SI; P10 S2, P7 S1*

This question appears to be concept-oriented or one that requires inference, but this is actually detail-oriented (i.e. mere recall of information). The correct answer, **C**, is a paraphrase of the definition provided in the second sentence of Paragraph 10: "a state where the values of the

macroscopic variables remain approximately stable." (Temperature and volume are examples of macroscopic variables as indicated in the first sentence of Paragraph 7.)

11. Question Type: _____
    Strategy: *SaL; P11*

This question mainly requires scanning and close attention to details. Each option slightly varies in wording, but the correct answer, **D**, is verbatim of the sentence in Paragraph 11 - "Kelvin's Second Law: There is no thermodynamic process whose sole effect is to transform heat extracted from a source at uniform temperature completely into work."

12. Question Type: _____
    Strategy: *SaL; P15 S2*

Although Clausius started introducing an earlier concept of "entropy" – the 'equivalence value' of a transformation – in 1854, he the coined the term in 1865 as indicated in the second sentence of Paragraph 15.

13. Question Type: _____
    Strategy: *SI; P15*

This is a concept-oriented question that requires you to first, understand the given concept and then apply or generalize it to real world situations.

Entropy, within the context of the author's discussion in Paragraph 15, involves variables transforming through a succession of equilibrium states and that the state of entropy increases. Among the given options, only the process described in **D** goes back (loop) to the initial stage of the system rather than transform to another equilibrium state. **D** is the EXCEPTION.

14. Question Type: _____
    Strategy: *SaL; P8 last two sentences*

"Statement and Reason" is another typical RC question in the DAT. The answer is commonly easy to locate through a simple scan of the passage. In this case, the information is found in the last two sentences of Paragraph 8.

A common decoy, however, is mixing up two different pieces of information from the passage, making the combination of the statement and its reason appear to be correct. The statement that "several mathematically exact approaches to thermodynamics now exist" is correct; but it was "rational thermodynamics" that helped clarify the concepts and logic of classical thermodynamics –NOT the other way around. Therefore, **(C)** the statement is correct but the reason is NOT.

15. Question Type: _____
    Strategy: *PoE; SaL*

This is another common type question in the DAT RC which can be classified as an "exception or negative question." Arriving at the correct answer entails scanning specific parts of the passage and eliminating true statements.

Statement A is supported by the third up to the last sentence of Paragraph 7 (P7 S3 to last sentence); Statement B by the second sentence of Paragraph 7 (P7 S2); Statement C by the fifth sentence of Paragraph 8 (P8 S5); and Statement E by the last sentence of Paragraph 7 (P7 last sentence).

Statement D expresses the reverse idea of the fourth sentence of Paragraph 7 (P7 S4). Clausius thought heat consisted solely of the motion of particles - WITHOUT an ether, NOT within the context of unobservable ether. **D** is the best answer.

16. Question Type: _____
    Strategy: *PoE, SaL, SI; P7 S1, P8 S2*

Answering this question requires you to combine SaL and evaluation of the concept of thermodynamics as discussed in the passage. The author states in the first sentence of Paragraph 7 that the variables of thermodynamics "range over macroscopic parameters such as temperature and volume." This eliminates options **A** and **B**. In the second sentence of Paragraph 8, macroscopic variables are also identified to be empirically adequate. Among options **C**, **D**, and **E**, only protons cannot be ordinarily observed. Therefore, **C** CANNOT be considered a variable in a thermodynamic process.

Would you like to discuss any of the answers
or strategies in this section?
Go to www.dat-prep.com/forum to share and learn.

GOLD STANDARD DAT RC PRACTICE TEST

Reading Comprehension Test

Time Limit: 60 Minutes

Passage 1

Scientific Analysis and Reasoning

(1). Unlike some other classical figures (Auguste Comte and Émile Durkheim, for example) Max Weber did not attempt, consciously, to create any specific set of rules governing social sciences in general, or sociology in particular. Compared to Durkheim and Marx, Weber was more focused on individuals and culture and this is clear in his methodology. Whereas Durkheim focused on the society, Weber concentrated on the individuals and their actions; and whereas Marx argued for the primacy of the material world over the world of ideas, Weber valued ideas as motivating actions of individuals, at least in the big picture.

(2). Weber was concerned with the question of objectivity and subjectivity. Weber distinguished social action from social behavior, noting that social action must be understood through how individuals subjectively relate to one another. Study of social action through interpretive means must be based upon understanding the subjective meaning and purpose that the individual attaches to their actions. Social actions may have easily identifiable and objective means, but much more subjective ends and the understanding of those ends by a scientist is subject to yet another layer of subjective understanding (that of the scientist). Weber noted that the importance of subjectiv-

ity in social sciences makes creation of full-proof, universal laws much more difficult than in natural sciences and that the amount of objective knowledge that social sciences may achieve is precariously limited. Overall, Weber supported the goal of objective science, but he noted that it is an unreachable goal – although one definitely worth striving for.

> *There is no absolutely "objective" scientific analysis of culture . . . All knowledge of cultural reality . . . is always knowledge from particular points of view . . . An "objective" analysis of cultural events, which proceeds according to the thesis that the ideal of science is the reduction of empirical reality to "laws," is meaningless. . . [because]. . . the knowledge of social laws is not knowledge of social reality but is rather one of the various aids used by our minds for attaining this end.*
>
> - Max Weber, "Objectivity" in ***Social Science,*** 1897

(3). The principle of "methodological individualism," which holds that social scientists should seek to understand collectivities (such as nations, cultures, governments, churches, corporations, etc.) solely as the result and the context of the actions of individual persons, can be traced to Weber, particularly to the first chapter of **Economy and Society**, in which he argues that only individuals "can be treated as agents in a course of subjectively understandable action." In other words, Weber argued that social phenomena can be understood scientifically only to the extent that they are captured by models of the behavior of purposeful individuals, models which Weber called "ideal types," from which actual historical events will necessarily deviate due to accidental and irrational factors. The analytical constructs of an ideal type never exist in reality, but provide objective benchmarks against which real-life constructs can be measured.

> We know of no scientifically ascertainable ideals. To be sure, that makes our efforts more arduous than in the past, since we are expected to create our ideals from within our breast in the very age of subjectivist culture.

- Max Weber, 1909

(4). Weber's methodology was developed in the context of a wider debate about methodology of social sciences, the *Methodenstreit* (debate over methods). Weber's position was close to historicism, as he understood social actions as being heavily tied to particular historical contexts and its analysis required the understanding of subjective motivations of individuals (social actors). Thus Weber's methodology emphasizes the use of comparative

historical analysis. Therefore, Weber was more interested in explaining how a certain outcome was the result of various historical processes rather than predicting an outcome of those processes in the future.

(5). Such views by Max Weber find their parallel in the field of twentieth-century scientific thoughts. Jacob Bronowski, writer of the book and the 1973 BBC television documentary series, **The Ascent of Man**, was a mathematician, biologist, historian of science, theatre author, poet and inventor. In the 1950s, he wrote an essay entitled *The Nature of Scientific Reasoning*, which similarly discusses subjectivity, this time among scientific theories, as the following excerpt would show:

(6). "No scientific theory is a collection of facts. It will not even do to call a theory true or false in the simple sense in which every fact is either so or not so. The Epicureans held that matter is made of atoms 2000 years ago and we are now tempted to say that their theory was true. But if we do so we confuse their notion of matter with our own. John Dalton in 1808 first saw the structure of matter as we do today, and what he took from the ancients was not their theory but something richer - their image: the atom. Much of what was in Dalton's mind was as vague as the Greek notion, and quite as mistaken. But he suddenly gave life to the new facts of chemistry and the ancient theory together, by fusing them to give what neither had: a coherent picture of how matter is linked and built up from different kinds of atoms. The act of fusion is the creative act.

(7). All science is the search for unity in hidden likenesses. The search may be on a grand scale, as in the modern theories which try to link the fields of gravitation and electromagnetism. But we do not need to be browbeaten by the scale of science. There are discoveries to be made by snatching a small likeness from the air too, if it is bold enough. In 1935, the Japanese physicist Hideki Yukawa wrote a paper which can still give heart to a young scientist. He took as his starting point the known fact that waves of light can sometimes behave as if they were separate pellets. From this he reasoned that the forces which hold the nucleus of an atom together might sometimes also be observed as if they were solid pellets. A schoolboy can see how thin Yukawa's analogy is, and his teacher would be severe with it. Yet Yukawa, without a blush, calculated the mass of the pellet he expected to see, and waited. He was right; his meson was found, and a range of other mesons, neither the existence nor the nature of which had been suspected before. The likeness had borne fruit.

(8). The scientist looks for order in the appearances of nature by exploring such likenesses. For order does not display itself of itself, if it can be said to be there at all, it is not there for the mere looking. There is no way of pointing a finger or camera at it; order must be discovered and, in a deep sense, it must be created. What we see, as we see it, is mere disorder.

(9). This point has been put trenchantly in a fable by Karl Popper. Suppose that someone wishes to give his whole life to science.

Suppose that he therefore sat down, pencil in hand, and for the next twenty, thirty, forty years recorded in notebook after notebook everything that he could observe. He may be supposed to leave out nothing: today's humidity, the racing results, the level of cosmic radiation and the stock market prices and the look of Mars, all would be there. He would have compiled the most careful record of nature that has ever been made; and, dying in the calm certainty of a life well-spent, he would of course leave his notebooks to the Royal Society. Would the Royal Society thank him for the treasure of a lifetime of observation? It would not. The Royal Society would treat his notebooks exactly as the English bishops have treated Joanna Southcott's box. It would refuse to open them at all, because it would know without looking that the notebooks contain only a jumble of disorderly and meaningless items."

- Part of this passage is adapted from J. Bronowski, *The Nature of Scientific Reasoning*

1. In the excerpt from Jacob Bronowski's essay, the author starts with "No scientific theory is a collection of facts." Which of the following reasons can NOT be inferred to be applicable to this statement?

   A. Theories are sometimes developed from other earlier theories.

   B. Facts from one era of history may differ from facts of later histories.

   C. Scientific theory can be a creative act through fusion of theories.

   D. Facts are immutable throughout time, while theories are not.

2. Weber's concept of methodological individualism is BEST exemplified by how one:

   A. conceives collective institutions as the product of individual actions.

   B. focuses on how social action can be understood through subjective interpretation.

   C. interprets "ideal types" on the basis of debate over methods.

   D. stands in stark contrast to social realities interpreted by Marx and Durkheim.

   E. represents as an agent in subjective social actions.

3. Jacob Bronowski is identified as all of the following EXCEPT a(n):

   A. mathematician.
   B. biologist.
   C. author.
   D. poet.
   E. philosopher.

4. The fable by Karl Popper can be inferred to express the idea that in scientific study:

   A. order must be discovered and created.

   B. a clear focus is needed to sort out the mess of variables.

   C. indiscriminate research findings will not be applauded by the scientific community.

   D. what we see, as we see it, is mere disorder.

   E. the Royal Society, in reality, regard scientific theories to be meaningless.

5. "Methodenstreit" means:

   A. methodology of social sciences.
   B. methodological individualism.
   C. debate over methods.
   D. scientific analysis and reasoning.
   E. social action.

6. According to Bronowski, science is characterized by a number of ideas. Which of the following is NOT an idea advanced in his essay?

    A. Science looks for order in the appearance of Nature.
    B. Science looks for unity in hidden likenesses.
    C. Science proceeds to build theory through testing and observation.
    D. Science is selective in its searches for order and likeness.

7. All knowledge of cultural reality is always knowledge from certain points of view.

    Social phenomena can be understood scientifically only to the extent that they are captured by "ideal types."

    A. Both statements are true.
    B. Both statements are false.
    C. The first statement is true. The second statement is false.
    D. The first statement is false. The second statement is true.

8. Hideki Yukawa discovered:

    A. that light waves could behave like pellets.
    B. the meson.
    C. that the nucleus of an atom was not held together similar to pellets.
    D. the link between gravitation and electromagnetism.
    E. that scientific theory is creative.

9. The notion of an objective scientific analysis of culture is unattainable because it will always be marked by subjective perspectives.

    A. Both the statement and reason are correct and related.
    B. Both the statement and the reason are correct but NOT related.
    C. The statement is correct but the reason is NOT.
    D. The statement is NOT correct, but the reason is correct.
    E. NEITHER the statement NOR the reason is correct.

10. Weber's opinion toward objectivity in the social sciences is that:

   A.   it is practically non-existent.
   B.   it is nothing more than an ideal.
   C.   it is masked by our very own subjectivity.
   D.   objective knowledge is limited.
   E.   it is more focused on individuals and culture.

11. Weber's "ideal types" are:

   A.   striving for objectivity through subjective means.
   B.   ideal methodologies for understanding social action.
   C.   socially-constructed realities based on subjective interpretation.
   D.   models of social behavior.
   E.   deviations due to accidental and irrational factors.

12. It can be inferred from the passage that "Methodenstreit" was:

   A.   a concern of how to properly define social action.
   B.   an argument of how to proceed theoretically in the study of social sciences.
   C.   a theoretical quagmire of evaluating objectivity.
   D.   a postulation of proof concerning subjectivity.

13. Which of the following concepts DOES NOT point out a difference of Weber from other classical figures in the social sciences?

   A.   Weber focused on individuals and their social actions.
   B.   Weber valued the ideas that drive individual actions.
   C.   Weber created standards albeit subjective for understanding society.
   D.   Weber was concerned with the question of objectivity and subjectivity.
   E.   Weber noted that social action must be understood through how individuals subjectively relate to one another.

14. Which of the following sociological studies would be reasonably expected to interest Weber?

   A.   A report on repercussions of President Bush's "War on Terrorism" policy
   B.   A subjective study of social behavior among victims of domestic violence
   C.   An analysis of Napoleon Bonaparte's motivation for waging the Napoleonic Wars
   D.   A research report on culture presenting the different findings and impressions of the researchers

15. According to Bronowski, the order of Nature must be:

A. discovered.
B. understood.
C. fused.
D. deduced.
E. debated.

16. Weber wrote the first chapter of *Economy and Society* in:

A. 1808.
B. 1897.
C. 1909.
D. 1935.
E. 1973.

17. The view that matter has primacy over ideas was promoted by:

A. Dalton.
B. the Epicureans.
C. Comte.
D. Marx.
E. Durkheim.

Passage 2

Drifting Rocks

(1). Another one of the devious little mysteries of science are the strange stones of Death Valley in California. These stones sit on sun-baked, flat, cracked earth, but for some baffling reason, they have moved across the wasteland. They have, in fact, left trails of their movement.

(2). The home of these mysterious stones is known, logically, as the "Racetrack Playa", a dry lakebed occasionally dampened by flash storms. The Racetrack measures 4.5 kilometers by 2.1 kilometers (2.8 by 1.3 miles), and is only about 5 centimeters (2 inches) higher at one end than the other.

(3). The trails left by the stones vary from a few meters to almost a kilometer in length. Some of the trails are straight; some are zigzagged; some go in circles. In some cases, the trails vary in width, meaning the stones must have rotated as they moved. One hundred sixty two of the Racetrack's moving stones have been documented, and many of them have names, always female. They range from fist-sized to the size of an ice chest.

(4). In 1948, two US Geological Survey geologists suggested that the little desert whirlwinds known as "dust devils" might be responsible for moving the stones around. Then George Stanley, a geologist of Fresno State College in California, suggested the stones might have become frozen in ice sheets during the winter and slid around with the sheets on an underlying slick of water.

(5). Between 1968 and 1975, two geologists, Robert Sharp of the California Institute of Technology and Dwight Carey of the University of California at Los Angeles, made careful measurements of the positions of 30 rocks in an attempt to answer the mystery of the drifting rocks once and for all. They tried to pound stakes around some of the rocks, on the principle that if the motion were caused by floating ice, the stakes would hold the ice in place. The mystery only seemed to deepen. In one case, a rock drifted out of the stakes while another remained where it was, and in other cases rocks moved near other rocks that remained stationary.

(6). Sharp and Carey never really managed to link the movement of a rock to any event and finally gave up. By this time, research has become somewhat restricted by the fact that the Racetrack is now a protected Wilderness area. The US National Park Service was trying to protect the Racetrack, which was suffering from increasing numbers of intruders who were not always considerate of the special nature of the place. Sometimes park rangers find citizens dancing naked on the dried mud, apparently obtaining inspiration from the place's cosmic energies. Drug runners also occasionally use it as a landing strip, though ranger vigilance has largely eliminated this practice. Rangers had to dig a trench to keep four-wheel drive vehicles out and kept the place tidied up.

(7). Meanwhile, researchers continue to puzzle over the drifting rocks. One early suggestion was that the rocks were driven by gravity, sliding down a gradual slope over a long period of time. But this theory was discounted when it was revealed that the northern end of the playa is actually several centimeters higher than the southern end and that most of the rocks were in fact traveling uphill.

(8). Nonetheless, John B. Reid, Jr. of Hampshire College in Amherst, Massachusetts, is a partisan of the ice floe theory while Paula Messina, assistant professor of geology at San Jose State University in California, thinks they move in the wind over a slick of mud when the Racetrack is wet. Reid does not buy the wind theory, basing his objections on studies performed by him and his students in the late 1980s and early 1990s, when they measured the force required to move some of the Racetrack's bigger rocks and determined that wind speeds of hundreds of kilometers per hour would be required to budge them – though it has been pointed out that Reid's measurements, taken in dry conditions, may not have accurately reflected what would happen when the Racetrack was wet.

(9). Though no one has yet been able to conclusively identify just what makes the rocks move, for the past ten years, Dr. Paula Messina has made it her quest to understand what has bewildered geologists for decades. "It's interesting that no one has seen them move, so I am kind of sleuthing to see what's really going on here," says Dr. Messina.

(10). Many scientists had dedicated much of their careers to the racing rocks, but the remoteness of the area kept their research limited in scope. No one had been able to map the complete set of trails before the advent of a quick, portable method known as global positioning. Dr. Messina was the first to have the luxury of this high technology at her fingertips.

(11). In 1996, armed with a hand-held GPS unit, she digitally mapped the location of each of the 162 rocks scattered over the playa. "I'm very fortunate that this technology was available at about the same time the Racetrack captured my interest," she says. "It took only ten days to map the entire network – a total of about 60 miles." Since then, she has continued to chart the movements of each rock within a centimeter of accuracy. Walking the length of a trail, she collects the longitude and latitude points of each, which snap into a line. She then takes her data back to the lab where she is able to analyze changes in the rocks' positions since her last visit.

(12). She has found that two components are essential to their movement: wind and water. The fierce winter storms that sweep down from the surrounding mountains carry plenty of both. The playa surface is made up of very fine clay sediments that become extremely slick when wet. "When you have pliable, wet, frictionless sediments and intense winds blowing through," offers Dr. Messina, "I think you have the elements to make the rocks move."

(13). At an elevation of 3,700 feet, strong winds can rake the playa at 70 miles per hour. But Dr. Messina is quick to point out that sometimes even smaller gusts can set the rocks in motion. The explanation for this lies in her theory, which links wind and water with yet another element: bacteria.

(14). After periods of rain, bacteria lying dormant on the playa begin to "come to." As they grow, long, hairlike filaments develop and

cause a slippery film to form on the surface. "Very rough surfaces would require great forces to move the lightest-weight rocks," she says. "But if the surface is exceptionally smooth, as would be expected from a bio-geologic film, even the heaviest rocks could be propelled by a small shove of the wind. I think of the Racetrack as being coated by Teflon, under those special conditions."

(15). In science, hypotheses are often based on logic. But over the years, Dr. Messina has discovered that on the Racetrack, logic itself must often be tossed to the wind. "Some of the rocks have done some very unusual things," she says. In her initial analysis, she hypothesized that given their weight, larger rocks would travel shorter distances and smaller, lighter rocks would sail on further, producing longer trails. It also seemed reasonable that the heavier, angular rocks would leave straighter trails and rounder rocks would move more erratically.

(16). What she discovered surprised her. "I was crunching numbers and found that there was absolutely no correlation between the size and shape of the rocks and their trails. There was no smoking gun, so this was one of the big mysteries to me." What appears as a very flat, uniform terrain is in fact a mosaic of microclimates. In the southeastern part of the playa, wind is channeled through a low pass in the mountains, forming a natural wind tunnel. This is where the longest, straightest trails are concentrated. In the central part of the playa, two natural wind tunnels converge from different directions, creating turbulence. It is in this area that the rock trails are the most convoluted. "What I think is happening," proposes Dr. Messina, "is that the surrounding topography is actually what is guiding the rocks and telling them where to go."

(17). Some people have suggested attaching radio transmitters to the rocks or erecting cameras to catch them "in the act" in order to put an end to the speculation. But as Death Valley National Park is 95 percent designated wilderness, all research in the park must be noninvasive. It is forbidden to erect any permanent structures or instrumentation. Further, no one is permitted on the playa when it is wet because each footprint would leave an indelible scar.

(18). As for Dr. Messina, she is content in the sleuthing. "People frequently ask me if I want to see the rocks in action and I can honestly answer that I do not," she says. "Science is all about the quest for knowledge, and not necessarily knowing all the answers. Part of the lure of this place is its mystery. It's fine with me if it remains that way."

- Adapted from "Drifting Rocks" (http://www.vectorsite.net/tamyst.html) Thanks to Greg Goebel.

18. The Racetrack Playa has an elevation of:

A. 5 centimeters.
B. 60 miles.
C. 10000 meters.
D. 3,700 feet.
E. 31,00 feet.

19. John B. Reid, Jr. believed in the same theory that George Stanley suggested in the late 1940s.

Robert Sharp and Dwight Carey disproved that the movement of the rocks was caused by floating ice.

A. Both statements are true.
B. Both statements are false.
C. The first sentence is true while the second sentence is false.
D. The first sentence is false while the second sentence is true.

20. In Messina's final hypothesis, she attributed the explanation behind the drifting rocks to be caused by:

A. bacteria-based slippery clay.
B. wind tunnels.
C. the terrain's topography.
D. ice floe.
E. mysterious forces.

21. The approximate sizes of the rocks have been described to range:

   A. from a few centimeters to 200 centimeters.
   B. from fist-sized to the size of an ice chest.
   C. from 100 centimeters up to a meter in size.
   D. from 200 centimeters up to 500 centimeters.
   E. The passage does not contain any description of size besides varied.

22. Suppose that Reid and his students were able to conduct their measurements in wet conditions with successful results. This would undermine another assertion made in the passage that:

   A. floating ice causes the movements of the rocks.
   B. the "dust devils" are causing the rocks to move.
   C. the stones, frozen in ice sheets during the winter, slide around with the sheets on an underlying slick of water.
   D. the wind is responsible for moving the stones over a slick of mud whenever the Racetrack is wet.

23. Winter storm winds come into the playa of up to:

   A. 80 mph gusts.
   B. 70 mph gusts.
   C. 90 mph gusts.
   D. 60 mph gusts.
   E. This information is not within the passage.

24. Dr. Messina's GPS unit has an x and y co-ordinate accuracy of:

   A. one centimeter.
   B. ten centimeters.
   C. five centimeters.
   D. twenty centimeters.
   E. This information is not contained in the passage.

25. How many drifting rocks are there in total?

   A. 126
   B. 30
   C. 162
   D. 261
   E. 612

26. The theory that the rocks were sliding down a gradual slope over a long period of time was proven to be true when it was revealed that wind speeds of hundreds of kilometers per hour would be required to budge them.

    A. Both the statement and reason are correct and related.
    B. Both the statement and the reason are correct but NOT related.
    C. The statement is correct but the reason is NOT.
    D. The statement is NOT correct, but the reason is correct.
    E. NEITHER the statement NOR the reason is correct.

27. Many of the moving stones in the Racetrack Playa have names which are:

    A. mythological.
    B. scientific.
    C. Native American.
    D. female.
    E. male.

28. Which of the following is the BEST reason that makes Dr. Messina's theory relatively strong?

    A. Limited variables
    B. Multiple causes
    C. Use of GPS
    D. Singular effects
    E. More accurate measurements

29. Reid's main contention with Messina concerning the drifting rocks concerns:

    A. ice.
    B. mud.
    C. direction.
    D. wind speed.
    E. trails.

30. Attaching radio transmitters to the rocks is not permitted on the Racetrack because rain or snow would negate any data collected from radios.

    A. Both the statement and reason are correct and related.
    B. Both the statement and the reason are correct but NOT related.
    C. The statement is correct but the reason is NOT.
    D. The statement is NOT correct, but the reason is correct.
    E. NEITHER the statement NOR the reason is correct.

31. Each of the following statements concerning Sharp and Carey is true EXCEPT one. Which one is the EXCEPTION?

A. They made careful measurements of 30 rocks on the Playa.

B. They used stakes to try to hold the rocks in place.

C. Both had insignificant and contradictory results.

D. Both are part of the US Geological Survey.

E. Both gave up in their research.

32. What Messina found from her GPS analysis was that:

A. wind tunnels of variable strength move the rocks around the slippery mud in a random pattern.

B. a combination of mud, slipperiness, wind, wet clay and bacteria account for the random distributions.

C. there was absolutely no correlation between the size and shape of the rocks and their trails.

D. the icefloe and dust devil theories could be ruled out based on trail positioning.

E. all prior theories lack the necessary GPS and computer analysis, therefore theoretically dubious.

33. Each of the following describes the rock trails EXCEPT one. Which one is the EXCEPTION?

A. Straight
B. Back and forth
C. Circling
D. Zigzagged
E. Varying in width

Passage 3

Forensic Dentistry

(1). Bite marks are an important and sometimes controversial aspect of forensic odontology. Forensic odontology is the study of dental applications in legal proceedings. The subject covers a wide variety of topics including individual identification, mass identification, and bite mark analysis. The study of odontology in a legal case can be a piece of incriminating evidence or an aspect of wide controversy. There have been many cases throughout history, which have made use of bite marks as evidence.

(2). Bite marks are usually seen in cases involving sexual assault, murder, and child abuse and can be a major factor in leading to a conviction. Biting is often a sign of the perpetrator seeking to degrade the victim while also achieving complete domination. Bite marks can be found anywhere on a body, particularly on soft, fleshy tissue such as the stomach or buttocks. In addition, bite marks can be found on objects present at the scene of a crime. Bite marks are commonly found on a suspect when a victim attempts to defend him or herself.

(3). Even though using bite mark evidence began around 1870, the first published account involving a conviction based on bite marks as evidence was in the case of Doyle v. State, which occurred in Texas in 1954. The bite mark in this case was on a piece of cheese found at the crime scene of a burglary. The defendant was later asked to bite another piece of cheese for comparison. A firearms examiner and a dentist evaluated the bite marks independently and both concluded that the marks were made by the same set of teeth. The conviction in this case set the stage for bite marks found on objects and skin to be used as evidence in future cases.

(4). Another landmark case was People v. Marx, which occurred in California in 1975. A woman was murdered by strangulation after being sexually assaulted. She was bitten several times on her nose. Walter Marx was identified as a suspect and dental impressions were made of his teeth. Impressions and photographs were also taken of the woman's injured nose. These samples along with other models and casts were evaluated using a variety of techniques, including two-dimensional and three-dimensional comparisons, and acetate overlays. Three experts testified that the bite marks on the woman's nose were indeed made by Marx, and he was convicted of voluntary manslaughter.

(5). Although there are many cases in which bite mark evidence has been critical to the conviction or exoneration of criminal defendants, there is continuing dispute over its interpretation and analysis.

(6). Factors that may affect the accuracy of bite mark identification include time-dependent changes of the bite mark on living bodies, effects of where the bite mark was found, damage on soft tissue, and similarities in dentition among individuals. Other factors include poor photography, impressions, or measurement of dentition characteristics.

(7). For bites on human skin, a potential bite injury must be recognized early, as the clarity and shape of the mark may change in a relatively short time in both living and dead victims. Bite marks most often appear as elliptical or round areas of contusion or abrasion, occasionally with associated indentations.

(8). Once the mark is initially evaluated, it should be examined by a forensic odontologist to determine if the dimensions and configuration are within human ranges. Since a large proportion of individuals (80-90%) secrete the ABO blood groups in their saliva, swabbing the area and a control area elsewhere on the body should be completed before the body is washed. Although there have been descriptions of using fingerprint dusting methods, photography is the primary means of recording and preserving the bite mark and is critically important in documenting the evidence. When there are indentations in the skin, or to preserve the three-dimensional nature of the bitten area, impressions should be taken to fabricate stone models. This is done by fabricating custom impression trays and taking an impression of the mark and surrounding skin with standard dental impression material. These impressions are then poured in dental stone to produce models. After the initial analysis is complete, there may be a need to preserve the actual skin bearing the mark. A ring of custom tray material can be made to fit like a hoop, closely approximating the skin, which can then be attached to the skin with cyanoacrylate adhesive and stabilized with sutures. When the pathologist completes the autopsy, the bite mark can be excised with the supporting framework in place.

(9). Studies have also been performed in an attempt to find the simplest, most efficient, and most reliable way of analyzing bite marks. Most bite mark analysis studies use porcine skin (pigskin), because it is comparable to the skin of a human, and it is considered unethical to bite a human for study in the United States. Limitations to the bite mark studies include differences in properties of pigskin compared to human skin and the technique of using simulated pressures to create bite marks. Although similar histologically, pigskin and human skin behave in dynamically different ways due to differences in elasticity. Furthermore, postmortem bites on nonhuman skin, such as those used in the experiments of Martin-de-las-Heras et al., display different patterns to those seen in antemortem bite injuries. In recognition of the limitations of their study, Kouble and Craig suggest using a G-clamp on an articulator in future studies to standardize the amount

of pressure used to produce experimental bite marks instead of applying manual pressure to models on pigskin. Future research and technological developments may help reduce the occurrence of such limitations.

(10). Kouble and Craig compared direct methods and indirect methods of bite mark analysis. In the past, the direct method compared a model of the suspect's teeth to a life-size photograph of the actual bite mark. In these experiments, direct comparisons were made between dental models and either photographs or "fingerprint powder lift-models." The "fingerprint powder lift" technique involves dusting the bitten skin with black fingerprint powder and using fingerprint tape to transfer the bite marks onto a sheet of acetate. Indirect methods involve the use of transparent overlays to record a suspect's biting edges. Transparent overlays are made by free-hand tracing the occlusal surfaces of a dental model onto an acetate sheet. When comparing the "fingerprint powder lift" technique against the photographs, the use of photographs resulted in higher scores determined by a modified version of the ABFO scoring guidelines. The use of transparent overlays is considered subjective and irreproducible because the tracing can be easily manipulated. On the other hand, photocopier-generated overlays where no tracing is used is considered to be the best method in matching the correct bite mark to the correct set of models without the use of computer imaging.

(11). While the photocopier-generated technique is sensitive, reliable, and inexpensive, new methods involving digital overlays have proven to be more accurate. Two recent technological developments include the 2D polyline method and the painting method. Both methods use Adobe Photoshop. Use of the 2D polyline method entails drawing straight lines between two fixed points in the arch and between incisal edges to indicate the tooth width. Use of the painting method entails coating the incisal edges of a dental model with red glossy paint and then photographing the model. Adobe Photoshop is then used to make measurements on the image. A total of 13 variables were used in analysis. Identification for both methods were based on canine-to-canine distance (1 variable), incisor width (4 variables), and rotational angles of the incisors (8 variables). The 2D polyline method relies heavily on accurate measurements, while the painting method depends on precise overlaying of the images. Although both methods were reliable, the 2D polyline method gave efficient and more objective results.

(12). Nevertheless, bite mark analysis is not without its critics. Recently, the scientific foundation of forensic odontology, and especially bite mark comparison, has been called into question. A 1999 study, frequently referenced in news stories but difficult to actually locate, by a member of the American Board of Forensic Odontology found a 63 percent rate of false identifications. However, the study was based on an informal workshop during an ABFO meeting, which many members did not consider a valid scientific setting.

(13). An investigative series by the Chicago Tribune entitled "Forensics under the Microscope" examined many forensic science disciplines to see if they truly deserve the air of infallibility that has come to surround them. The investigators concluded that bite mark comparison is always subjective and no standards for comparison have been accepted across the field. The journalists discovered that no rigorous experimentation has been conducted to determine error rates for bite mark comparison, a key part of the scientific method. Critics of bite mark comparison cite the case of Ray Krone, an Arizona man convicted of murder on bite mark evidence left on a woman's breast. DNA evidence later implicated another man and Krone was released from prison. Similarly, Roy Brown was convicted of murder due in part to bite mark evidence, and freed after DNA testing of the saliva left in the bite wounds matched someone else.

- Portions of this passage are adapted from "Experimental Studies of Forensic Odontology to Aid in the Identification Process" by Susmita Saxena, Preeti Sharma, and Nitin Gupta. *Journal of Forensic Dental Sciences*, 2010 Jul-Dec; 2(2): 69–76.

34. Recent investigation into bite mark analysis shows that this procedure suffers from:

    A. a shortage of methods to actually quantify the identification of a person's teeth.
    B. a lack of rigorous experimentation to determine error rates.
    C. failure to follow the scientific method at a paradigmatic level.
    D. a lack of willing research associates, concerned with such analysis.
    E. a shortage of replication studies, to help confirm analysis results.

35. A 1999 study claims a bite mark false identification rate of:

    A. 36%.
    B. 33%.
    C. 63%.
    D. 66%.
    E. The passage does not indicate this information.

36. Each of the following is a factor that may affect the accuracy of bite mark identification EXCEPT one. Which one is the EXCEPTION?

    A. Time-dependent changes of the bite mark on living bodies
    B. Effects of where the bite mark was found
    C. Damage on soft tissue
    D. Jaw alignment ratios in proportion to dental symmetry
    E. Poor photography, impressions, or measurement of dentition characteristics

37. Which of the following sentences would be the best conclusion for the closing paragraph?

A. When reporting on bite mark evidence, dentists should be transparent about the inherent obstacles to accurate analysis.

B. Despite issues on the accuracy of bite mark analysis procedures, several legal precedents allow for the admissibility of such evidence.

C. Indeed, an opinion is worth nothing unless the evidence is clearly describable and accurate when presented in court.

D. After all, bite mark analysis has almost non-existent valid rules, regulations, or processes for accreditation to standardize the evidence they provide in court.

E. Despite dentistry being a scientific field, forensic odontology remains a subjective science prone to errors.

38. Of the 2D polyline method of identification, which of the following set of variables used in analysis is correct?

A. Canine-to-canine distance (2 variables), incisor width (3 variables), and rotational angles of the incisors (8 variables)

B. Canine-to-canine distance (1 variable), incisor width (4 variables), and rotational angles of the incisors (8 variables)

C. Canine-to-canine distance (1 variable), incisor width (8 variables), and rotational angles of the incisors (4 variables)

D. Canine-to-canine distance (4 variables), incisor width (1 variable), and rotational angles of the incisors (8 variables)

E. Canine-to-canine distance (8 variables), incisor width (1 variable), and rotational angles of the incisors (4 variables)

39. A direct method of identification would be the "fingerprint powder lift" technique.

An indirect method of identification would be the use of transparent overlays.

A. Both statements are true.
B. Both statements are false.
C. The first statement is true.
The second statement is false.
D. The first statement is false.
The second statement is true.

40. Which of the following methods do Kouble and Craig suggest to address the problems posed with the use of pigskin in bite mark analysis?

    A. Experimenting with other animal forms such as cows or horses to determine error rates

    B. Using a G-clamp manipulator to increase the standard intensity of pressure used

    C. Using a comparison of both direct and indirect methods in relation to pressure used

    D. Using a G-clamp on an articulator to standardize the amount of pressure used

    E. Keeping the pigskin at the same temperature as the victim kept in the forensic lab

41. Forensic odontology was first publicly recognized in:

    A. 1780.
    B. 1954.
    C. 1975.
    D. 1945.
    E. 1870.

42. Each of the following is a legal proceeding concerning bite mark identification mentioned in the passage EXCEPT one. Which one is the EXCEPTION?

    A. Manslaughter
    B. Kidnapping
    C. Child Abuse
    D. Sexual Abuse
    E. Burglary

43. Suppose an investigator is skeptical over the bite mark evidence presented against a murder suspect. How would a forensic odontoligst BEST convince the investigator that the procedure performed is reliable?

    A. Bite marks found on the victim's body were deep, indicating that the act was deliberate and premeditated.

    B. A second set of dental impressions was obtained from the suspect himself.

    C. The autopsy was performed 24 hours after the crime was committed.

    D. The marked area was swabbed for traces of saliva and submitted for DNA testing.

    E. Photocopier-generated overlays were employed to match the murderer's correct bite mark.

44. Which of the following persons was convicted of burglary based on bite mark evidence left on a piece of cheese?

A. Marx
B. Krone
C. Doyle
D. Brown
E. Martin-de-las-Heras

45. The use of transparent overlays is considered subjective and irreproducible because there are differences between pigskin and human skin.

A. Both the statement and reason are correct and related.
B. Both the statement and the reason are correct but NOT related.
C. The statement is correct but the reason is NOT.
D. The statement is NOT correct, but the reason is correct.
E. NEITHER the statement NOR the reason is correct.

46. What is The BEST method for bite mark analysis to date?

A. Transparent overlays
B. Photography
C. Fingerprint dusting
D. 2D polyline method
E. Painting method

47. The 2D polyline method employs Adobe Photoshop in bite mark analysis identification.

The painting method uses AUTOCAD in bite mark analysis identification.

A. The first statement is true, while the second statement is false.
B. The first statement is false, while the second statement is true.
C. Both statements are true.
D. Both statements are false.
E. There is not enough information within the passage to make a judgment.

48. ABFO stands for:

A. American Board of Forensic Odontologists.
B. American Board of Forensic Odontology.
C. Associated Board for Forensic Odontology.
D. Associated Board of Forensic Odontologists.
E. American Board for Forensic Odontology.

49. Each of the following bite mark analysis techniques were used in the case of the People vs. Marx EXCEPT one. Which one is the EXCEPTION?

A. Acetate overlays
B. Two dimensional comparisons
C. The "fingerprint lift method"
D. Three dimensional comparisons
E. Other models and casts

50. The experiments of Martin-de-las-Heras et al., found that:

A. the use of G-Clamp on an articulator standardized the amount of pressure in bite mark analysis.
B. postmortem bites on nonhuman skin displayed the same patterns as antemortem bites.
C. transparent overlays and tracing could easily be sketched in error.
D. postmortem bites on nonhuman skin displayed different patterns from antemortem bites.
E. the 2D polyline method without tracing is the most efficient method to date.

If time remains, you may review your work. If your allotted time (60 minutes) is complete, please proceed to the Answer Key.

Practice Test 1 Answer Key

1. D	18. D	35. C
2. A	19. C	36. D
3. E	20. C	37. B
4. A	21. B	38. B
5. C	22. B	39. A
6. C	23. B	40. D
7. A	24. A	41. B
8. B	25. C	42. B
9. A	26. E	43. D
10. B	27. D	44. C
11. D	28. B	45. B
12. B	29. D	46. D
13. C	30. C	47. A
14. C	31. D	48. B
15. A	32. C	49. C
16. C	33. B	50. D
17. D	34. B	

Practice Test 1 Explanations and Strategies

1. Answer: D
    Question Type: *Exception/Negative Question; Evaluation Question (Main Idea)*
    Strategies: *SI, PoE; P6*

    This question requires a careful inference of the basic premises of an author's view. By using the process of elimination, the correct statements can be inferred and are mentioned in Paragraph 6. D, being the exception, is the correct answer, which is supported by the phrase "which every fact is either so or not so" in Sentence 2 of Paragraph 6.

2. Answer: A
    Question Type: *Evaluation Question (Implication)*
    Strategies: *SI, paraphrasing, never lose sight of the question; P3 S1*

This is another inference question that requires you to carefully understand the essence of a theoretical concept. All options are mentioned in the passage at one point or another. Thus you need to remain focused on what the question is truly asking, which can be found in the first sentence of Paragraph 3: "The principle of 'methodological individualism,' which holds that social scientists should seek to understand collectivities (such as nations, cultures, governments, churches, corporations, etc.) solely as the result and the context of the actions of individual persons. . ."

3. Answer: E
    Question Type: *Exception/Negative Question*
    Strategy: *SaL; P5 S2*

4. Answer: A
    Question Type: *Evaluation Question (Main Idea)*
    Strategies: *SI, inference; P8*

    Although D is close and a direct quote in the passage, it is the preceding quote in that penultimate paragraph which provides the best answer (A) stating, "The scientist looks for order in the appearances of nature by exploring such likenesses. For order does not display itself of itself, if it can be said to be there at all, it is not there for the mere looking. There is no way of pointing a finger or camera at it; order must be discovered and, in a deep sense, it must be created". We cannot just infer D and leave it at that, but infer that the answer to this disorder is through discovery and creation of order, from the jumble of appearance. The fable is supposed to illustrate this preceding

idea.

The other answers are also partially correct but lack the overall explanatory power of A.

5. Answer: C
    Question Type: *Recall*
    Strategy: *SaL; P4 S1*

6. Answer: C
    Question Type: *Exception/Negative Question*
    Strategies: *SaL, inference; P7, P8*

    A, B and D are ideas advanced by Bronowski as can be found in the following, respectively: P8 S1, P7 S1, and P8 S2. He never mentions theory-building through testing and observation, even though one could infer that this method underlies "science."

7. Answer: A
    Question Type: *True or False Statements*
    Strategy: *SaL; P2 S2 of quoted paragraph; P3 S2*

8. Answer: B
    Question Type: *Evaluation (Implication)*
    Strategies: *SI, inference, prior knowledge; P7 S10*

    The answer to this question can be tricky unless you are familiar with the subject from prior knowledge. This is because Yukawa's discovery is presented in the passage in narrative form rather than as a straightforward description. Hence you need to be careful in reading the paragraph where this is discussed (P7) in order to infer the correct answer.

"Yukawa, without a blush, calculated the mass of the pellet he expected to see, and waited. He was right; his meson was found, and a range of other mesons, neither the existence nor the nature of which had been suspected before."
The other statements are corollaries, hypotheses, or distractions.

9. Answer: A
    Question Type: *True or False Statements (Statement and Reason)*
    Strategy: *SI; P2 quoted paragraph*

    The answer is supported by Weber's own quote:

    "There is no absolutely 'objective' scientific analysis of culture... All knowledge of cultural reality... is always knowledge from particular points of view."

    Here, "particular points of view" expresses "perspective."

10. Answer: B
    Question Type: *Evaluation Question (Main idea)*
    Strategies: *SI, inference; P2 last sentence and quoted paragraph*

    This question requires a keen understanding of the gist of Weber's view on objectivity in the social sciences. This can be best inferred in Paragraph 2 as follows:

    "Overall, Weber supported the goal of objective science, but he noted that it is an unreachable goal – although one definitely worth striving for. . . An 'objective' analysis of cultural events,

which proceeds according to the thesis that the ideal of science is the reduction of empirical reality to 'laws,' is meaningless. . . [because]. . . the knowledge of social laws is not knowledge of social reality but is rather one of the various aids used by our minds for attaining this end."

11. Answer: D
    Question Type: *Recall*
    Strategy: *SI; P3 S2*

    "In other words, Weber argued that social phenomena can be understood scientifically only to the extent that they are captured by models of the behavior of purposeful individuals, models which Weber called 'ideal types.'"

12. Answer: B
    Question Type: *Evaluation Question (Main Idea)*
    Strategies: *SI, inference; P4 S1*

    This question requires you to deduce the meaning of the term in question in its paraphrased form. A, C, and D are partially correct, but only to the extent that they can be included in B, meaning any debate about methodology used in a given discipline or science, is one that sets up standards for the proper theoretical approach – or how to proceed theoretically, in adopting a methodology for the study.

13. Answer: C
   Question type: *Recall*
   Strategy: *SI; P1 and P2*

   C is the opposite of the idea expressed in Sentence 1 of Paragraph 1. The rest are either verbatim or can be inferred from Paragraphs 1 and 2.

14. Answer: C
   Question Type: *Application Question*
   Strategies: *SI, inference; P4 S3*

   The answer to this question cannot be found in an exact statement in the passage. However, you are required to use the information provided in the passage as basis for evaluating the given options.

   Paragraph 4 of the passage makes clear that Weber is more concerned in studying the motivating factors of individual actions, rather than in determining the effect of such actions: "Weber's methodology emphasizes the use of comparative historical analysis. Therefore, Weber was more interested in explaining how a certain outcome was the result of various historical processes rather than predicting an outcome of those processes in the future."
   Option C obviously complements Weber's methodology.

15. Answer: A
   Question Type: *Recall*
   Strategy: *SaL; P8 S3*

16. Answer: C
   Question Type: *Recall*
   Strategy: *SaL; P3 S1 and quoted paragraph*

17. Answer: D
   Question Type: *Recall*
   Strategy: *SaL; P1 last sentence*

18. Answer: D
   Question Type: *Recall*
   Strategy: *SaL; P13 S1*

19. Answer: C
   Question Type: *True or False Statements (Two Statements)*
   Strategies: *SI, attention to details; P4 S2*

   The statements given in this question are paraphrased from different parts of the passage. This requires locating the relevant paragraphs and then inferring the main ideas.

   The first statement is derived from information contained in Paragraph 4 Sentence 2 and Paragraph 8 Sentence 1. Essentially, both George Stanley in the late 1940s and John B. Reid, Jr. in the 80s and 90s attributed the movement of the rocks to the floating ice sheets.

   The second statement is derived from the last two sentences of Paragraph 5 and Sentence 1 of Paragraph 6. Although Sharp and Carey were not able to prove anything, nothing was also conclusive in the measurements they conducted.

20. Answer: C
    Question Type: *Recall*
    Strategy: *SaL; P16 S1*

21. Answer: B
    Question Type: *Recall*
    Strategy: *SaL; P3 last sentence*

22. Answer: B
    Question Type: *Application Question*
    Strategies: *OA, inference; P8 S2, P13 S1*

This question requires that you infer the implications behind the theories brought forward in the passage.

In Paragraph 8, although Reid was able to discount the factor of the wind in the rocks' movements, results of his study were only based on dry conditions. This still leaves the possibility of the wind being a factor in the drifting rocks phenomenon during the wet weather.

On the other hand, had Reid's findings been proven consistent on wet conditions, this might even give more credit to the floating ice theory as the wind would be eliminated as a contributing factor in the rocks' movements in ANY condition. This eliminates option A.

B cannot be the best answer because "dust devils" only occur on dry conditions. Results derived from dry conditions are already enough to discount the "dust devils" as the driving force behind the drifting rocks.

C is also wrong. The statement in this option has nothing to do with the contention about the wind as a factor in the rocks' movements.

This leaves D as the most possible answer. According to Reid's study, "wind speeds of hundreds of kilometers per hour would be required to budge (the rocks)." In Paragraph 13, strong winds are measured to yield a force of only 70 miles per hour.

23. Answer: B
    Question Type: *Recall*
    Strategy: *SaL; P13 S1*

24. Answer: A
    Question Type: *Recall*
    Strategy: *SI; P11 S4*

25. Answer: C
    Question Type: *Recall*
    Strategy: *SaL; P3 S3*

26. Answer: E
    Question Type: *True or False Statements (Statement and Reason)*
    Strategies: *SaL, inference; P7 S2 and S3, P8 S2*

The information given in this question is almost verbatim of certain parts in the passage. What is tricky here is that the first statement is obviously wrong. Paragraph 7 indeed explains that the theory of the rocks sliding down a gradual slope due to gravity was discounted when it was discovered that the rocks were in fact traveling uphill. On the other hand, the second statement is true as indicated in

Paragraph 8. However, Reid's conclusion about the wind speeds has more to do with the wind and the "dust devil" theories and does not have a direct link to the rock's sliding movement. Hence, this bit of information is still an incorrect reason in relation to the gravity theory. This makes (E) neither the statement NOR the reason correct.

27. Answer: D
Question Type: *Recall*
Strategy: *SaL; P3 S3*

28. Answer: B
Question Type: *Evaluation Question (Implication)*
Strategies: *OA, inference; P6 S1, P8, P10 to P16*

It must be noted that the other researchers who conducted measurements in the Playa either failed to prove anything or focused on only one possible cause of the rocks' movements.

Sharp and Carey never really managed to link the movement of a rock to any event and finally gave up.

John Reid was able to disprove the wind theory but ironically did not come up with a proof to support the ice floe theory.

On the other hand, Messina conducted several observations for a span of ten years to trace the cause behind the "drifting rocks" mystery. Rightfully so for a subject as complex and variable as the rocks in the Playa, Dr. Messina came up with a number of plausible explanations as denoted in Paragraphs 12, 13, and 16.

29. Answer: D
Question Type: *Recall*
Strategy: *SaL; P8 S1*

30. Answer: C
Question Type: *True or False Statement (Statement and Reason)*
Strategy: *SaL; P17*

31. Answer: D
Question Type: *Exception/Negative Question*
Strategy: *SaL; P4 S1, P5, P6 S1*

Option A is supported by Sentence 1 of Paragraph 5, Option B by Sentence 2, and Option C by the last two sentences. Option E is also supported by Sentence 1 of Paragraph 6. On the other hand, the two geologists from US Geological Survey were never named in Sentence 1 of Paragraph 4 while Sharp and Carey were clearly identified with California Institute of Technology and University of California at Los Angeles, respectively.

32. Answer: C
Question Type: *Recall*
Strategy: *SaL; P16 S1*

33. Answer: B
Question Type: *Recall*
Strategy: *SaL; P3 S2 S3*

34. Answer: B
Question Type: *Recall*
Strategies: *SI, attention to details; P13 S3*

35. Answer: C
Question Type: *Recall*
Strategy: *SaL; P12 S3*

36. Answer: D
Question Type: *Exception/Negative Question*
Strategy: *SaL; P6*

"Jaw alignment ratios in proportion to dental symmetry" does not constitute "similarities in dentition among individuals."

37. Answer: B
Question Type: *Evaluation Question (Main Idea)*
Strategy: *OA; P1, P3, P4, P10, P11, P12*

This question requires your overall understanding of the passage's main message. By looking at significant clues in the different paragraphs, you will realize that the main purpose of the author is to illustrate that despite the various contentions on the methods used in bite mark analysis, they all boil down to the fact that the evidence they bring about is after all, admissible in court.

This is clearly conveyed from the beginning of the passage (P1 last two sentences): "The study of odontology in a legal case can be a piece of incriminating evidence or an aspect of wide controversy. There have been many cases throughout history, which have made use of bite marks as evidence." The last sentence of Paragraph 3 further supports this view stating, "The conviction in this case set the stage for bite marks found on objects and skin to be used as evidence in future cases."

While the statement in A sounds ideal, no specific part in the passage indicates the author advocating this view.

C is obviously off on a tangent.

Option D is countered by Paragraph 10 Sentence 7 in defense of standardization of the bite marks analysis procedure: "the use of photographs resulted in higher scores determined by a modified version of the ABFO scoring guidelines."

Option E can likewise be contended by the fact that the passage presented scientific methods used in bite mark evidence and oppositions were made mostly by journalists (non-scientific). The 1999 study cited in Sentence 3 of Paragraph 12 also casts doubt to the real persona (and hence credibility) of the member of the American Board of Forensic Odontology who was "frequently referenced in news stories but difficult to actually locate."

38. Answer: B
Question Type: *Recall*
Strategy: *SaL; P11 S7*

39. Answer: A
Question Type: *Recall*
Strategy: *SaL; P10 S3, S5*

40. Answer: D
Question Type: *Recall*
Strategies: *SaL, attention to details; P9 S6*

41. Answer: B
    Question Type: *Recall*
    Strategies: *SaL, never lose sight of the question; P3 S1*

    This question can be tricky, and you have to be careful in identifying that what is being asked is the date when forensic odontology (dental applications in legal proceedings) was first publicly recognized. This could have only been possible with the publication of the case of Doyle v. State in 1954.

42. Answer: B
    Question Type: *Recall*
    Strategies: *SaL, attention to details; P2 S1, P3 S2, P4 last sentence*

43. Answer: D
    Question Type: *Application Question*
    Strategies: *SI or OA, attention to details; P8 S2, P13*

    This question can be easily answered if you have been paying close attention to the information presented in the last paragraph of the passage. It should be noted that the significant evidence that reversed the court's sentences to Krone and Brown was DNA testing. Swabbing of the saliva specimen, which is essential in DNA testing, in bite mark analysis procedure is further supported by Sentence 2 of Paragraph 8.

    Option A is quite subjective and therefore, not convincing. Option B is a plausible method to confirm a dental match of a suspect; so is E. However, a DNA match still qualifies

as stronger evidence. C describes one of the factors affecting the accuracy of bite mark analysis. The best answer is D.

44. Answer: C
    Question Type: *Recall*
    Strategy: *SaL; P3*

45. Answer: B
    Question Type: *True or False Statements (Statement and Reason)*
    Strategies: *SI, inference; P9 S4, P10 S8*

    A quick review of Paragraphs 9 and 10 would prove that both the statement and reason in this question convey correct information. However, the reason for the use of transparent overlays being subjective and irreproducible is because the tracing can be easily manipulated. Thus, the reason given in the question is not related.

46. Answer: D
    Question Type: *Recall*
    Strategies: *SaL, PoE, attention to details; P11 last sentence*

    Reviewing the last sentence of Paragraph 11 would help eliminate option E. Sentence 8 of Paragraph 10 likewise negates option A as the correct answer. Sentence 3 Paragraph 8 indicates (C) Fingerprint dusting as merely one of the methods and (B) photography as the primary means - not the best method - of recording and preserving bite marks. This leaves D as the best answer.

47. Answer: A
    Question Type: *True or False Statements (Two Statements)*
    Strategy: *SaL; P11 S3*

48. Answer: B
    Question Type: *Recall*
    Strategies: *SaL, attention to details; P12 S3*

49. Answer: C
    Question Type: *Recall*
    Strategies: *SaL, attention to details; P4*

50. Answer: D
    Question Type: *Recall*
    Strategies: *SI, inference; P9 S5*

> Would you like to discuss any of the answers
> or strategies in this test?
> Go to www.dat-prep.com/forum to share and learn.